BREASTLESSNESS

BREASTLESSNESS

A Journey of Faith and Empowerment After a Breast Cancer Diagnosis

What To Do When You Don't Know What To Do

M. Nicole Bryant

PRECISELY WRITE PUBLISHING
East Carondelet, IL

PRECISELY WRITE PUBLISHING
P. O. Box 411
East Carondelet, IL 62240

©2005 by M. Nicole Bryant

All rights reserved. This book is protected under the copyright laws of the United States of America. No part of this book may be reproduced or transmitted in any form or by any means, electronic or mechanical, including photocopying, recording or by any information storage or retrieval system without written permission, except where permitted by law.

ISBN: 0-9778612-0-1
Library of Congress Control Number: 2006901510

Edited by Linda S. Lawson
Cover and Interior Design by Al Nichols
Author Photograph by Suzy Gorman
Production by Messenger Printing Co., Inc.

ATTENTION CORPORATIONS, UNIVERSITIES, COLLEGES, CLINICS, AND PROFESSIONAL ORGANIZATIONS: Quantity discounts on bulk purchases of this book are available. Book excerpts can also be created to fit specific needs. For information, please contact Precisely Write Publishing, P.O. Box 411, East Carondelet, IL 62240; phone 618-286-3648.

Printed in the United States of America

AN IMPORTANT NOTE

This book is meant to inspire, uplift, educate, and empower. It should not be used as a substitute for care by a qualified medical professional or health care provider. It is intended to provide information to assist the reader in understanding the medical information and advice offered by her/his physician and to help the reader participate in decisions that affect her/his well-being and health.

The author and publisher have made every attempt to ensure that the information presented is accurate up to the time of publication. However, due to ongoing breast cancer research, it is possible that new findings may invalidate some of the data presented here. We assume no responsibility for errors, inaccuracies, omissions, or any inconsistencies herein.

The names of some of those involved have been changed to protect their privacy and identities.

My Lord and Savior Jesus Christ

You are worthy to be praised; for You are an awesome God. I give You all the honor, glory, and praise. My continued health is a testimony of the power of prayer, and of your loving kindness, grace, and mercy. Unto Thee, O God, I give thanks. Thank You for loving me when I sometimes didn't love myself. You said in Your word that you would never leave or forsake me. Thank You for keeping my mind, body and spirit in perfect peace. I am humbled by my daily blessings of life and good health.

Dedication

<u>To my daughter, Michelle, and granddaughters, Briannah, Jerica and Urie</u>

You were the source of my strength and courage during this crisis. You are the reason I fought (and still fight) so hard to beat this disease. Fighting became easier when I kept you in my mind and my heart. The thought of leaving you wouldn't allow me to give in or give up. My life has been so enriched by all of you. Because of my diagnosis and that of your dad's sister, you are at an increased risk of getting this disease. It is my prayer that you be spared this legacy; I will do all within my power to eradicate such a fate. May God continue to bless you with good health. The poet Elizabeth Barrett Browning wrote it best: *"I love you to the depth, height and breadth my soul can reach."*

Acknowledgments

Many, many thanks to Anita Payne and Wendy Weiner for their assistance in preparing the very first draft of this manuscript in 1997.

Linda Lawson who lent her skillful writing to the editing process. Her professionalism, patience, and commitment were invaluable.

Al Nichols whose input and creative contributions to this project are deeply appreciated.

Christine Frank for contributing her talent, skill, and insight.

Gratitude and many thanks to the American Cancer Society for permission in using its unlimited resource material.

Special expressions of gratitude to Mary Hunt and Karen Fryberger of Positive Promotions and Kim Klonower of Cooper Surgical for the use of their illustrations.

To my dedicated team of proofreaders, Michelle, Katina, Heather, Marsha, Hannah, and Jacqueline. Thanks for unselfishly giving so much of their time to this project.

A. Janine Coleman for her commitment in seeing this project through.

HONORABLE MENTIONS

Please indulge me for I have a lot of people to thank for the place I now stand.

My Mother

Thank you for embracing me with your love and your strength. You gave me that which I could never give you—life, and for that I'm profoundly thankful. Thank you for praying for me when I wasn't praying for myself. Your guidance helped mold and shape me into the person that I am. I love you. I miss you. Your legacy of strength, compassion, and courage lives through me.

My Son, Julius

I don't know if there are any words in the English language to explain how I feel about you or powerful enough to express how much you mean to me. Thank you for being so supportive during those first months of my diagnosis and subsequent surgeries. Thanks for all the Chinese food. I love you.

My Sisters and Brothers

All of you were very instrumental in my recovery and in helping me to appreciate the importance of having your family stand beside you in a crisis. Your support gives testimony that love is stronger than any hardship or crisis. Through this experience, you helped me re-appreciate the power of laughter, the strength of the human spirit, and the lesson to never take little things for granted. There were a lot of times when I felt like giving up, but your love and prayers kept me going. I love you, and may God continue to bless and keep you. Thank you, Barbara, Johnnie, Dorothy, Jesse, Michael, Evelyn, Sharon, Sheena, and Angela.

My Very Special Friend

George, you were there when I was first diagnosed and you were there through all my surgeries and my recoveries. You were there during the good, the bad, and the ugly times. Thanks for taking such good care of me when I wasn't able to take care of myself. I know that it was more than a notion for you and for that I will be forever grateful. You are a dear friend, a very special man and a wonderful human being. May God continue to bless you.

My D.C. Connection

Even though I was a complete stranger to you, you were kind enough to share your wisdom, your experience, and your love. Had it not been for you, I would not have learned how to fight for my life. Thank you, Gillie.

My California Connection

My sincere thanks for your support and prayers, and allowing me to express my fears, my sadness, my laughter, and every new experience with you. You played a big part in getting me back to me. To my friends Barbara (Jean) Dixon, Marsha Pinkard-Jackson, Jacqueline Alfred-Kranson, Dena Hurst-Semmons, Katrin Spinetta, Heather Thompson, Richard Williams, Wanna Wright, and KyungBin Yi.

To the doctors, nurses, CNAs, lab technicians, and staff at Kaiser Hospital, Oakland, California, especially Dr. June George. Thank you for taking such good care of me.

A debt of gratitude to Jackie Pugh and all the staff and members of the American Cancer Society's Reach To Recovery Program, Women's Cancer Resource Center, the Charlotte Maxwell Complimentary Clinic, Oakland, California, and Alta Bates Comprehensive Breast Cancer

Center, Berkeley, California. You gave me (and countless others like me) hope through your expressions of love, support, and compassion. You contributed greatly to my emotional and physical well-being, keeping me sane during an otherwise insane period in my life. Thank you for allowing me to participate in and be a part of such worthwhile, valuable and needed programs.

My Illinois Connection

To the Pastor and members of Flat Creek Missionary Baptist Church. Thank you for being such committed and faithful prayer warriors.

To Charles and Helen Johnson. I can't thank you enough for the countless times you came to my rescue. May God continue to bless you.

Hannah Brown, Patricia Brewer, and Tom Edwards. God has blessed me by putting some very special people in my life…people like you who are strong, caring, prayerful, purposeful, and willing to share all that God has given. Thank you for keeping me motivated and focused. Thank you for all your support, advice, and encouragement.

To Sharon Bills and Sharon Stepney. Thanks for supporting my dream.

My Missouri Connection

To the staff of Barnes-Jewish Hospital/Washington University, Breast Health Center in St. Louis. Thank you for consistently providing quality care not only to me but to all cancer patients.

CONTENTS

Acknowledgements..v
Honorable Mentions..vi
Introduction...x

PART ONE

1	What's Breasts Got to Do With It?	3
2	The Diagnosis…My Journey Begins	18
3	Devastated But Not Destroyed	34
4	The Emancipation of My Symbol of Beauty	48
5	One Titty Gone	63
6	The Phantom Breast Blues	72
7	Beyond The Shadows	83
8	Whose Breasts Are These Anyway?	91
9	Still On My Journey	108

PART TWO

10	Dispelling The Myths; Understanding the Facts	121
11	Know Your Breasts	129
12	Screening And Warning Signs	140
13	Breast Cancer Treatment Options	166
14	Ask Questions…Then Ask More Questions	192
15	Just For Men	210
16	Know Your Rights; You Have a Right To Know	216
17	Where To Go, Who To Call	229
18	Words You Need To Know	240

Resources & References	270
Index	272
About the Author	277

INTRODUCTION

According to the American Cancer Society, nearly 185,000 women were diagnosed with breast cancer in 1994. This statistic meant nothing to me; that is, until I became one of them that year. I was living a myth; one that so many of us find ourselves living without even knowing it. I didn't associate this disease with women of color. Like so many other ailments, I foolishly thought that breast cancer wasn't mine to have. I didn't know just how at risk I was. If anyone had told me twelve years ago that I would be one of those women, a statistic, I would have thought they were crazy or at least delusional. Little did I know that my chances of being diagnosed with breast cancer were far greater than I could have ever imagined. I was uninformed, unconcerned, and unprepared.

Before this became "my disease," I never thought about breast cancer—I had no reason to think about it. It was just something I thought affected only white women. I didn't know anyone with the disease and had only personally known one other person who had died from cancer. I vaguely recall seeing a commercial or two on TV, but nothing that affected my world enough to get my attention. I don't recall reading any articles about the disease. And yes, I have at some point in my life subscribed to *Ebony, Essence, Jet, Cosmopolitan, Working Woman, Working Mother, Time and Newsweek*, and to my local newspaper. I watched *Oprah, 60 Minutes, 20/20, Dateline, Primetime*, the evening news, and even watched a few health programs on the cable networks. I no doubt missed the segments or just plain ignored the articles when breast cancer was featured.

I'd heard of only one other African American woman who had been diagnosed with breast cancer. In 1979, Minnie Riperton, a very talented and beautiful songstress, died of the disease at age thirty-one. Even then, I could not relate to Ms. Riperton or equate this ailment to African American women because it appeared to me to be an isolated and rare incident. No alarms sounded, no red flags were raised for me. There were no magazine articles or news programs that told the stories of countless other African American women who died from the disease.

Nor did I see stories that told the successes of women who lived to tell other African American women of their triumph.

In 1979, I was twenty-seven. The thought of my health being compromised never crossed my mind. It took nearly fifteen years for me to equate this disease with another African American woman —me.

I tragically learned there were many other women whose bodies betrayed them. Looking for answers, I searched for anything that would help me to understand how this could happen. I needed to know that there were others with whom I could identify. What I realize now is there are countless women in my same predicament, or even worse. I also realize my lack of concern was probably in part because I didn't see faces like mine representing this disease.

Since my return to the Midwest from California, I've discovered the statistics are no better here than they were there. Women in the Midwest, particularly African American women, are also dying from breast cancer. When I contemplated the message I wanted this book to convey, I reflected upon my diagnosis, treatment, and concerns. I was worried about everything…my health, my family, my job, and my mortality. I needed to know there were others who shared my health crisis, and lived. I needed to know what, if anything, I could do to help myself. Most importantly, I needed to know that a future was possible and I would live to see my grandchildren become adults.

My original thought was to just write a story about me, and how I dealt with the circumstances of my life. I realized that just telling my story wasn't enough; my responsibility to other women required more than that. I needed to write something that would have a long-lasting and positive impact on the lives of the women (and men) who read this book. I hope the reader appreciates it for its candor and embraces it because of its potential to make a difference in someone's life, maybe even to save a life. I believe anyone who has been faced with a potentially life ending disease can relate to my story; however, it is especially important to me that women of color have something, someone they can identify with, learn from, and be empowered by.

Several years after my diagnosis, while going through some old papers, I found two physicians' referral slips for me to have a mammography exam. One was scheduled for April and another in July. I'm embarrassed to say that I cancelled both of them. I don't know what I was doing in April or July of 1993 that would have been more important than keeping those appointments. In any event, not one professional contacted me about the cancelled appointments. It wasn't as if I had been told that I *should* have the mammogram. No one seemed overly concerned; so consequently, I wasn't concerned either. I now realize that my health care was just as much or more my responsibility than it was that of the doctors.

I know now that nothing could have been more important than my health or my life. Someone asked me if I had kept those mammography appointments, would my outcome have been different. It would not have changed the diagnosis, but it could have possibly changed my treatment option. A woman shared with me that she hadn't gone for a mammography because she heard the procedure hurts. I showed her a picture of me with one breast. "THIS hurts!" I'd rather have a thousand mammograms than to have one cancer diagnosis. The momentary discomfort doesn't hurt nearly as much as rounds of chemo, rounds of radiation, or rounds of regret. I can't say it enough. It can't be stressed enough. It can't be repeated enough. Early detection, diagnosis and treatment save lives. It saved mine; it can save yours!

If one grandmother, mother, sister, daughter, aunt, and yes, father, son, brother, or husband reads my words and finds they have helped her/him cope or empower them in some way, then my goal has been accomplished. If my circumstances should, by chance, bring comfort to someone who might not know that a breast cancer diagnosis doesn't necessarily mean the end of one's life or living a full life, then I've done a good job. And, if my story brings someone to God or back to Him, then I've done an exceptional job…the job I was meant to do.

This book is divided into two parts. ***Part One, "Breatlessness,"*** is about me. It's a very honest and intimate story about my journey before, during, and after my diagnosis. I talk candidly about my discovery, diagnosis, subsequent surgeries, and issues with this new body. I discuss healing from the physical and emotional scars, how I was able to focus on what breast cancer brought to my life rather than what it took away, and how I was able to accept and make peace with having this disease.

Part Two, "What To Do When You Don't Know What To Do," was written solely with you in mind. This section, above all else, is intended to educate, enlighten, and empower you. It provides you with enough information so you can make informed and realistic decisions about your health care. The decisions you make will play an important role in your well-being. Hopefully, some of the mistakes I made can be avoided. I've tried to cover everything a person should know before making a choice.

You are faced with some many anxieties when diagnosed with this disease. The last thing you want to do is have to search for information about it and figure out what you need to do next. This section is literally a one-stop information center. If you discovered a lump on your breast would you ignore it? Would you know what to do? What if you didn't have a regular doctor or have any insurance, would you know where to go for help? Would you know what to ask the doctor or better yet, would you know if you were getting the best care possible? You will have to make many decisions; you will encounter things that you weren't prepared for. This section will help with the navigation so that you, along with the advice of your doctor(s), can do what you feel is best for optimum health and overall well-being.

I pray that my story will serve as a beacon of hope to countless individuals who need it and send a resounding message that we don't have to die. I hope that by sharing my story the secrecy, guilt, and stigma associated with this disease will be removed.

The American Cancer Society estimates that nearly 200,000 women will be diagnosed with breast cancer in 2006. Statistics are merely numbers until a name and face are associated with them. Someone you love, someone you know, maybe even you, will be one of these women or men—a statistic. Being diagnosed with breast cancer is like preparing for battle. Battling the disease is like fighting a formidable war. Don't be just a statistic; don't be just a causality of this war. Be armed, engaged, and equipped to win.

"A wise man should consider that health is the greatest of all human blessings."

Hypocrites

PART ONE

About Me

BREASTLESSNESS
A Journey of Faith and Empowerment After a Breast Cancer Diagnosis

Early Diagnosis and Treatment Can Save Your Life

To My Sisters United By Faith

To women everywhere of every race, creed, color, and nationality. Every grandmother, mother, daughter, sister, wife, aunt and friend who has been diagnosed with this disease. May my life be a symbol of hope and a source of inspiration.

1
What's Breasts Got To Do With It?

My breasts always had a mind of their own. They did what they wanted, when they wanted, whether I liked it or not. They grew when they got good and ready; sagged (somewhat) when I didn't want them to. They aided in my sexuality without my permission. Sometimes, my breasts weren't so kind to me, but then again, I haven't always been particularly nice to them either. Without my knowledge or giving me advance warning, they held my life in their bosom. They have been nipped, tucked, cut, removed, reduced, and reconstructed (some by choice, others by necessity). One or more of the procedures could easily describe my love/hate relationship with my breasts. Collectively they played a major role in how I was able to cope with my body image, how profoundly my life was changed by breast cancer, and facing my mortality.

I'm still perplexed by why we place so much emphasis on them. In our obsession to achieve the quintessential illusion of perfect breasts we've been "lifted and separated," given "just our size," and have been made to feel "wonderful" and " angelic" by an array of lace, underwire, seamless, strapless, backless, cupless, wireless, see-through, push-up, padded, long line, and "cross your heart" bras.

The perfection of breasts have lifted egos, boosted the economy, and created more controversy than ever. Young women opt for bigger breasts, while mature women want perky ones. We stampede to plastic surgeons in our quest to make our breasts look more youthful, firmer, and better. We are told that bigger is better; that size matters. We've been misled to believe that our sexuality and our beauty are somehow inextricably associated with them. I'm the first to admit that I too was misled.

While I didn't get their mystique, I have learned they are a very powerful phenomenon. Breasts (or the lack of them) have caused marriages to end, relationships to suffer, and been instrumental in the sale of everything from Pepsis to Porsches. They cause men to grovel, young boys to fantasize, and women to feel both insecure and powerful.

Early Diagnosis and Treatment Can Save Your Life

There appears to be no end to the allure of the female breasts. They have been the subject of more articles than any other body part. There's even a Hollywood movie about their revolution. Breasts have been called everything from tits, boobs, hooters, jugs, melons, and cream puffs (as mine were). They have been used to feed our babies and satisfy our men. They have been heralded as defining our womanhood; yet, have been the source of so much of our pain and anguish. I read an article where a tribe of Amazon women would cut off one of their breasts as a symbol of their strength and courage. My experience wasn't quite that barbaric or symbolic. Nevertheless, having my breast removed did, ironically, serve as a catalyst in reclaiming my inner strength and the courage to fight for my life.

Breast cancer has been both a blessing and a curse. It made me take stock of my priorities, my insecurities, and yes, my life. Along the way to my diagnosis, I lost sight of what genuine beauty was. It's ironic my breasts would ultimately help me put things in proper perspective. My breasts didn't make me sexy nor did they make me whole. It is my love for me and my love for life that makes me do my proud peacock strut. I now realize just how blessed I am. I know, as I did prior to breast cancer, that beauty, femininity, and wholeness have absolutely nothing to do with body parts, particularly the size and shape of one's breasts.

Getting through the many phases of my physical development has been a journey in and of itself. Before I learned to appreciate what God gave me, I had to go through some things.

My Adolescence and Teens

My first recollection regarding breasts wasn't even about my own. It was the Mothers of the church who occupied the first two pews on the left side of the sanctuary. Mother Peterson, Mother Belt, Mother Nixon, Mother Charles, and my grandmother, Mother Rose, all looked the same shape and size. When they sat down, their breasts sat in their laps. Their arms rested gently across them as if they were extensions of their breasts. I automatically assumed that when you got old your breasts mushroomed as large as theirs. They didn't appear to serve any purpose and just seemed to be in the way. When you're young and flat chested, all breasts appear super-sized. I

Early Diagnosis and Treatment Can Save Your Life

knew even then that I didn't want them, ever!

I was thirteen and in junior high school when I first started paying attention to my own. I was somewhat ambiguous and indifferent about them; not particularly liking them, but not disliking them either. I frankly didn't understand why they were given to us in the first place. They were no big deal except they were a part of my body. What I did notice was mine were considerably smaller than those of most of the other girls my age, and they were especially smaller than those of two of my older sisters.

My oldest sister Barbara, who was three years older than I, developed early. Back then, I considered her the black Dolly Parton. Mother Nature had been extremely generous to her. No pills, no implants, no surgeries. She possessed what I thought were the largest breasts I'd ever seen on a sixteen-year-old girl. It may not have been they were so large as much as they stuck out more than most. On Barbara's thin frame, her breasts protruded like two large missile warheads. If launched, they could obliterate an entire country. They were pulled up very high, almost under her chin. I didn't know if that was the way breasts were supposed to sit or if it was the way she wore them. No matter what type of bra she wore (which usually was those one-of-a-kind ugly white bras with the thick straps, just like my mother's), her breasts announced her arrival.

Even though my sister Dorothy was just one year older than I, she was totally developed by the time she was fourteen. I mean developed. She had a bodacious body to carry those breasts. They looked as if Picasso, on his best day, painted the most flawless specimens on her chest. They were so firm, perfectly shaped, as if carved and sculpted just for her. No matter what she wore, it looked as if her breasts were a part of the clothing and not her body. And, if my memory serves me correctly, she had that body when she was twelve. I used to hear folks say that country girls developed faster. Well, the fresh air, the good country living, my mamma's good cooking, and all that running and playing didn't have the same effect on me.

I couldn't understand how Mother Nature could do such a wonderful job on Dorothy, and fail so miserably with me. How could she get breasts and a body like that, especially since we were just a year apart? It just seemed unfair. While the younger boys always acted so silly when she came around, the older boys seemed to want to devour her. I didn't understand

Early Diagnosis and Treatment Can Save Your Life

what this strange power was that she had over them. Little did I know, but some of that power, if not all of it, were in her bosom. I hoped that I would develop into a carbon copy of her. It didn't happen.

I waited, and waited, and waited while Mother Nature took her own sweet time. Almost daily, I would peek down my blouse hoping she would work her magic on me, praying there would be a significant change in their size. There wasn't. Dorothy's "perfect" breasts seemed to just appear on her chest overnight. I wanted mine to do the same. I watched, hoped, and prayed. Needless to say, nothing happened for a long time. Not only did Mother Nature take an eternity with me, but also when she did kick in, I wasn't pleased at all with the outcome. I was about fifteen when I finally start to "bud" as my mother called it. No one noticed them. Mine didn't get the same reaction as Dorothy's. I am not sure if I wanted that kind of attention, but it certainly would have helped to at least be acknowledged for my growth.

Women with large, eye-catching breasts surrounded me. One of my cousins, whose breasts were three times the size of mine, teased me a lot. Mine even got their own nickname, cream puffs. And if the size of my breasts wasn't bad enough, one of them looked different. The nipple on my left breast didn't protrude, as if it was turned inside out. I was very self-conscious about it and would discreetly look at the breasts of the other girls. None of them, white or African American, in the entire ninth grade gym class had breasts like mine. I wasn't perverted or anything, I just knew that mine looked different and I didn't understand why. I would rather die than let anyone see it. I was careful to shield my body when I undressed, showered, and put on my clothes. I just wanted to get through high school without anyone noticing that it was deformed. I wanted breasts like every other girl in school. Better yet, I wanted mine to be just like my sister's.

I thought my situation was hopeless. I figured Mother Nature had done all she was going to do with me. Not only were my breasts small, but I didn't have a big butt either. My sisters constantly teased me.

"You have a butt like a white girl," they would tease me.

"God gave you a big butt, and all you can do is sit on it. At least He gave me brains," I proudly boasted.

I was always quick-witted to mask my insecurities. I couldn't do anything about my butt; my breasts were a different matter. I had a few options in mind. I thought about wearing a padded bra. That would have meant sharing my feelings with my mother because she had to purchase it. Talking to my mother about my breasts wasn't going to happen. I even considered stuffing panties or thick bobby socks in my bra. While this seemed like a novel approach, it wasn't very practical or sensible. I chose to do neither; however, I was convinced there had to be a solution out there somewhere to fix my situation.

In addition to all my other problems, my oily skin caused terrible bouts with acne. For a sistah to have small breasts, no butt, and bad acne was not a good combination. I was, or so I thought, never going to be "pretty," nor was I ever going to like the way I looked. While most of my anxieties stemmed from my insecurities and hang-ups about my breasts, I eventually started feeling insecure about my entire physical appearance. There were no magazine articles at the time that told me I was a black butterfly waiting to spread my wings.

At sixteen, my prayers were answered. I found boob heaven in a Frederick's of Hollywood catalog nestled in my mother's drawer. It would solve most, if not all, my breast problems and then some. Not only could I buy padded bras that would make me appear to have larger breasts, but I could buy underwear that would give me a bigger butt, too. Even though I knew wearing a padded bra made absolutely no sense, I still felt the need to look like everyone else. I knew that some of my white classmates were wearing them and they were pleased, so it must be okay for me.

I wouldn't dare let my mother know what I was contemplating. I decided that I wanted my own copy of the catalog and immediately sent for my subscription. I could order my bits and pieces in secret. When my first copy arrived a few weeks later, I was completely engrossed in what one could purchase. The four-inch heels, the lingerie, the risqué clothing, and most of all, the selection of bras and undergarments were all way too mature for a sixteen year old. However, they were just the things I thought I needed and was determined to have.

Despite receiving several issues, I didn't muster the nerve to order anything. It could have had something to do with the fact that I didn't have any money, and there was just something unnatural or 'un-black' about all the fake stuff. Not to mention my biggest fear that sooner or later someone

Early Diagnosis and Treatment Can Save Your Life

would have discovered my secret anyway, or even worse, the pads would fall out during gym class.

I thought things could not get any worse, but then I had even bigger concerns. Hair began to grow on my chest and my calves seemed to be larger than most of the other girls. After reading a magazine article about a woman who suffered from a hormonal imbalance and developed male features, I just knew this was me. This woman grew facial and body hair, acquired a deeper voice, her once-shapely legs became muscular and her shoulders became broader. My overactive imagination had me believing that somehow I was changing into a boy. It appeared I was experiencing some of the same symptoms.

Some days it looked as if the hair on my chest was getting longer and thicker and my breasts were shrinking. I convinced myself this had to be the reason my left breast was different and why they weren't getting bigger. The possibility of becoming a boy was absolutely horrifying. I just knew it was only a matter of time before I would no longer be a girl. I prayed this wasn't going to happen to me. I never shared my concerns with anyone, secretly living in fear that Mother Nature had played another cruel trick on me, and my mother.

Time passed and instead of changing into a boy, Mother Nature changed tactics. I discovered boys, or should I say a young man discovered me. By the time I was seventeen, I was pregnant with my first child. I was the oldest child at home, and already playing the role of surrogate mother to some of my six younger siblings. Playing mother was challenging enough at seventeen; I didn't expect to become one. My mother never discussed sex at all. The only thing I clearly remember her saying was to keep my dress down and my legs closed. Unfortunately for me, I didn't quite get the meaning of that until it was too late. A look into my eyes told my mother I was pregnant before I knew. It was then we had our "talk." By then, the damage was done. Consequently, instead of our first serious talk being about the birds and the bees, we discussed babies and bottles.

One of the early signs of my pregnancy was that my little breasts started increasing in size. She told me they were growing because of the milk they produced. She forgot to tell me that once all the milk was gone, they would decrease in size, returning to their initial "cream puffs."

Early Diagnosis and Treatment Can Save Your Life

While I certainly wasn't ready for motherhood, maybe I could at least reap some of its benefits—larger breasts. Well, unlike most women, my breasts didn't get much larger than they had been prior to my pregnancy. By the time my baby was born, they had grown to a whopping 36B! I was now faced with the decision to breast-feed or not. I wanted to go back to school; how would I feed my baby while there? Pregnant girls were barely allowed to go to school, so I knew taking a baby there was completely out of the question. I was determined to graduate and, thank God, my mother was even more so. Consequently, breast-feeding was an absolute no-no for me. Furthermore, I was pleased with my new look, and didn't want to the chance of them shrinking too quickly. Bring me the bottle, where's the Similac, put the pacifier in his mouth, anything but my breasts.

Following my son's birth, my constant worry became whether they would sag. In an attempt to prevent it, I slept in my bra all the time. Seventeen should not be the age you worry about whether your breasts are going to sag. When you're young the only things that really matter is that you want to be cute, you want to be liked by your peers, you want to have fun, and you want to look like and be anybody else other than yourself.

My Twenties

The day before my twentieth birthday, I was given my daughter as a present. It was the beginning of me really establishing my own identity and feeling as if I were an adult away from home and the protective comfort of my mother. By age twenty-three, I had my own place, a job, and was attending a local university. I was pretty independent for a single mother with two children, and considered myself somewhat sophisticated and savvy. Everything I knew about taking care of myself and raising my babies, I got from my mother. Everything I'd learned, or that I thought I knew about being uninhibited, charming, and in control, I'd gotten from *Cosmopolitan Magazine* and those risqué romance novels by Danielle Steel.

Along the way, I now developed a new sense of self-confidence and a different attitude. I now liked the body I inhabited, and especially liked my small breasts. Even after two children, I managed to keep my shape and my breasts remained firm. Small breasts were "in" so I felt very comfortable

Early Diagnosis and Treatment Can Save Your Life

with the ones I had. I could wear those cute little tops. No bra. Had a little cleavage. Even thought I had a little sex appeal. Young men began to pay attention to me and I took pleasure in this new-found popularity. They seemed to be both fascinated and curious about me. I'm really not sure if it were my breasts drawing attention or something subtler that I didn't recognize. I was beginning to understand the power of sexuality.

At the time, I started dating one of the most popular young men on campus. I was captivated by him and thrilled to death he was interested in the little country girl from East Carondelet. Anthony was especially fond of my small breasts and I was especially glad that he was fond of them. For the first time, I actually enjoyed having them fondled. It didn't bother me so much anymore that my left one was different. I quickly learned what made the boys act so silly around my sister Dorothy. No matter how small they are, how big they are, or the shape—men like breasts!

In the fall of 1975, I moved from East St. Louis, Illinois to Oakland, California. I quickly discovered Californians were more conscious of their bodies, their skin, their hair, their nails, their feet, their teeth, and yes, their breasts. Just when I thought I had conquered most of my mammary demons, my insecure feelings resurfaced. Besides, I was in California where all the "beautiful people" were, and there was a doctor in the Bay Area who could fix almost any imagined or real imperfection. One could get long nails like Cher, hair like Diana Ross, a nose like Lena Horne, a smile like Farrah Fawcett, and yes, breasts like Dorothy's.

I finally learned that the nipple on my left breast wasn't deformed; it was inverted. I decided I was going to do something about it. Size didn't concern me anymore. I wanted better breasts; more specifically, I wanted a better nipple on my left breast. I don't know how or when I came to the decision to consult a plastic surgeon, but I do know I was almost obsessed with fixing it.

During the summer of 1976, I landed a job at an architectural firm in the Financial District of downtown San Francisco, located equally in distance from Union Square and Embarcadero Center. Both areas were very cosmopolitan, peppered with lots of upscale boutiques, hair salons, fine clothing stores like Neiman Marcus, I Magnin, and Saks, restaurants, outdoor cafes, and what became my favorite spot, Shaw's Shoes. And yes, there were a

Early Diagnosis and Treatment Can Save Your Life

multitude of doctors' offices. Needless to say, I spent the majority of my lunch time in and out of the stores on Maiden Lane near Union Square and clothing stores at the Embarcadero Center. The times when I was not in the boutiques, I was going in and out of plastic surgeon's offices picking up medical brochures with "before" and "after" photos. I was hopelessly enraptured by the glamour of San Francisco.

While window shopping and browsing through stores in Union Square, I saw a poster that piqued my fascination. It was an advertisement for breast augmentation. If this doctor could make breasts larger, certainly there was one who could fix my nipple. Once again, I found answered prayers in the quest for perfect breasts.

Having no idea where to find this miracle worker, I did the next best thing—I looked in the Yellow Pages. I don't even know what I based my decision on when I finally picked the plastic surgeon. As far as I knew, one was just as good as the next. Plastic surgery wasn't very popular, affordable, or accessible to African Americans. I didn't care. I was about to make a dream of mine come true. I would not only get the nipple I always wanted, but I would get nicer breasts in the process, like those in the magazines.

My appointment to see the plastic surgeon was during my lunch hour. Prior to my visit, I didn't do any reading or research about cosmetic surgery. I was excited about the possibility of having my nipple corrected, but was also apprehensive because I knew absolutely nothing about the procedure I was contemplating. I was willing to chance almost anything.

I followed the tall blond woman into an examination room. She gave me a long white gown in which to change.

"You can undress from the waist up," she instructed. "The doctor will be with you momentarily."

The doctor and the nurse entered the room. The nurse carried a tray that contained what looked like plastic pouches full of clear Jell-O. Each one varied in size and shape. As the doctor examined me, I wondered why males dominated those medical fields dealing with female issues (Pap smears, delivering babies, cosmetic surgery). I felt very uncomfortable having this strange white man touching my breasts. I

Early Diagnosis and Treatment Can Save Your Life

wished I had chosen a woman. I tried to relax, hoping the doctor wouldn't detect how uncomfortable I was. I did very little talking, partly because I didn't know what to ask, and mostly because I felt so out of place.

The gel-like pouches on the tray were silicone implants. I suspect they were the choice of the day and the answer for small-breasted women everywhere who felt they needed them. The purpose of my visit was to obtain information about correcting my inverted nipple. The doctor tried to convince me it was bigger breasts that I needed.

The exam and consultation took less than an hour; however, it seemed much longer.

"You can get dressed now, Ms. Bryant," the nurse finally said.

The doctor and nurse walked out and I began to dress.

"What the hell are you doing?" I thought. I was more confused when I left the doctor's office than when I arrived. I didn't want bigger breasts. I wanted better breasts. And more than anything, I wanted a better nipple!

I arrived back to work just as my lunch hour ended. I sat at my desk pondering why I would even consider such a procedure. Why had I felt so strongly about having perfect breasts? Besides, my body and my breasts held their own, considering I had birthed two children. I convinced myself I needed them. I didn't want a smaller waistline, a bigger butt, longer hair, not even prettier skin. I just wanted to look in the mirror and experience perfection. I knew I should have been thankful for the body God gave me and just leave well enough alone.

Finally, my good sense returned and I opted not to have the surgery. I would leave my breasts and my nipple as they were. As my thirties approached, I conquered all my breast demons. I was happy with life and matured into what I would like to think was a fairly grounded individual. I was working for a prestigious engineering firm, was having fun, and living life passionately. My experiences had been more than could be imagined for a small town girl. I was at peace with myself. None of my accomplishments, successes, disappointments, or failures had anything to do with my body or my breasts.

Early Diagnosis and Treatment Can Save Your Life

My Thirties

While on medical leave from injuries I sustained in an elevator accident, I met George, who was affectionately called Big G by his family and friends. I was thirty-five. He was forty-six. While I wasn't looking for a relationship, one quickly developed. George was one of those men who liked to cook and did it very well. Talk about being spoiled. He cooked breakfast almost every Saturday and Sunday morning, which I ate in bed. George would have dinner prepared for me when I arrived home from classes at 9:30 at night. All I had to do was eat, which I usually did while in bed. Our favorite daily dessert was Häagen Dazs Macadamia Nut Ice Cream. And no, we couldn't share—I had to have my own half pint, and he his own half pint. All that good loving and good cooking packed on the pounds. Before I knew it, I was wearing a 40D bra. When I met George my breasts were still a nice size and I could still go without a bra. Now, I was overweight with two large footballs on my chest, looking more and more like my sister, Barbara.

The luxury of bralessness and wearing just about anything was gone. I had to purchase new bras. To my surprise, the larger the breasts, the more the bra cost, and my choices were limited. They just weren't making the really cute lacy ones in larger sizes. Also gone were the slim hips and small waistline. I dealt with the expanding waist and hips pretty well. I could wear clothes to camouflage them. My breasts, on the other hand, were another matter. Large breasts could not be hidden or made to appear smaller.

By my late thirties, I was probably closer to one half pint of Häagen Dazs away from that 40DD than I cared to admit. I tried to justify the extra flesh hanging over my bra as cleavage. Buying a DD cup bra was completely out of the question, so I continued my denial wearing bras too small and blouses too large.

For such a long time I prayed for my breasts to be bigger. Then I wished they were better. And while I wanted them to be different, I didn't expect the change to be so drastic. I never would have imagined they could balloon so. My mammoth breasts presented new challenges when shopping for clothes. Jackets and blazers became an important part of my wardrobe because I could use them to cover up. If I purchased a

Early Diagnosis and Treatment Can Save Your Life

two-piece outfit, I always had to switch the top. While I could still fit into a size 12 skirt or pants, I was wearing a size 16, and sometimes 18 blouse, depending on the style and fabric. It was time to depart with a lot of the cute little things of old.

I had now gained about twenty-five pounds since I'd met George and fifteen of those went straight to my chest. I begrudgingly accepted my large breasts, but accepting them did not mean I liked them. There were many times when I wished they were small again. The bigger my breasts got, the larger the areola got, the more pronounced my inverted nipple became. I prayed that if I gained another pound it would go to my butt. To my dismay, it didn't. At some point, I finally reconciled that my body changes were due in part to my heritage. My chest was beginning to look more and more like my grandmother's.

In 1991, I worked with a young girl named Renee whose breasts were so abnormally large that I didn't know they carried bras in those letters. I thought Barbara's were big, but hers were small compared to Renee's. She complained constantly about how bad her back and shoulders hurt because of them. Just looking at them made my shoulders hurt. Renee eventually had breast reduction surgery. When I saw the results, I was amazed at the difference. The doctors did a wonderful job. She now looked normal, her breasts in proportion to her body. Mine were going to be next if they grew another inch.

My Forties

It goes without saying that most of my forties were spent taking care of my breasts instead of caring about them. I'd spent so much time worrying about what they looked liked, what I wished they looked like, whether they would sag, how little they were, how big they had become. All the attention I gave them would take on new meaning.

My forties would bring a profound change in my life that ironically involved my breasts. They would ultimately play a pivotal role in redefining my image of me and my outlook on life. Not only were they the source of my pain, anxiety, and fear, but also the catalyst for my physical, emotional, and spiritual growth.

Early Diagnosis and Treatment Can Save Your Life

What's Breasts Got To Do With It?

In June of 1994, at the age of forty-two, I discovered a lump in my left breast; the very breast that had given me so much grief for most of my life. Everything that I had done, felt, or thought about my breasts now seemed trivial—they then became my enemy. Breast cancer made an unwelcome and unexpected intrusion into my life, forcing me to switch gears.

In one instant, those carefree days, the "I'll do it tomorrow," and the promise for my future seemed to evaporate. Or at least I thought.
Once again I found myself in the unenviable position of having this tug of war between them and me. I found myself, again, watching other women's breasts. I envied them. I wanted what they had.

I recognized that in order to heal, I had to accept my body was never going to be the way it once was. Time has a way of making things right and healing wounded spirits. I was real clear about my breasts and what they have to do with it…everything and nothing. It took me a while, but I finally got it! My breasts meant ***everything*** in terms of my physical health, emotional well-being, and my survival. They meant ***nothing*** in terms of my inner beauty, strength, and my self-worth. My breasts did not validate me as a woman–they never did. Body parts don't make you who you are, but for a while, particularly after the mastectomy, I allowed myself to believe that. Breast cancer has a way of making you crazy, if only temporarily.

I realized I couldn't help others before helping myself. I recognized that in order to heal, I had to accept my body was never going to be the way it once was. There were so many times when I felt guilty and angry about having this disease. I never considered myself a victim nor did I act like one, but I was at the lowest point of my life. I needed to find some way to completely heal this vessel that housed my spirit as well as my soul. I relied heavily on my faith and prayed that I would be okay. One step at a time, one day at a time, I began my road to not just surviving, but thriving. And eventually, things changed, but the change I initially hoped for wasn't quite what I got.

There were times when I foolishly thought that I had been tested enough, and things couldn't get any worse. I survived a lot of challenges and most of the not-so-nice stuff life unexpectedly threw at me.

Early Diagnosis and Treatment Can Save Your Life

What I didn't know was God was just getting started with me. Breast cancer shook me to my core, making me lose a lot of things. It did not, however, make me lose my faith.

Breast cancer was my way of reclaiming my life and finding my way back to God. Every experience, every tear, every joy, every test of my faith was God's way of preparing me for something miraculous—for such a time as this.

Early Diagnosis and Treatment Can Save Your Life

> *I will praise thee: for I am fearfully and wonderfully made: marvelous are thy works; and that my soul knoweth well.*
>
> **Psalm 139:14**

2

The Diagnosis...My Journey Begins

My descent into emotional hell began with my witnessing the murder of two people. Then, my first grandchild, Eric, died of SIDS at three months old. Shortly thereafter, my apartment caught on fire. Due to work shortage, the land surveying company where I was employed laid me off—twice in a three-year period. In June of 1992, my best friend's (Jo) mother died. In October of 1992, Jo died. My aunt's homegoing was in November of 1993. In April of 1994, AIDS took the life of my youngest brother, Milton. In between, several more friends and friends' children passed. I had lost a lot; I'd been through a lot. I had been tested enough. I was wrong.

Jo's death affected me especially hard; it was very sudden and a complete surprise. For a long time I was angry at God for taking her. She was just too good of a person, too unselfish, too giving and too caring to die. Jo and I had been best friends since we were fourteen and fifteen, respectively. We grew up together, went to college together, partied together, and moved to California together. We held similar jobs as marketing coordinators for engineering firms. She was there when my granddaughter was born and cut the umbilical cord. Likewise, I was in the delivery room when her first grandson was born. We couldn't be any more bonded than Siamese twins. I cried every single day for the first year following her death. I missed our friendship, her compassion for others, and her ability to make anyone she came into contact with feel loved. God truly must have needed an angel to take her. I just wished He had chosen someone else and not my friend.

On top of all the other stuff, my son needed an exorcism. Without going into details, let's just say the bail bondsman and I were on a first name basis. My life had also been in turmoil. A lot of times I felt helpless, emotionally drained, and I know I was spiritually lost. I cried so much that I really felt there were no more tears to shed for anything or anybody. I had nothing left to give. I found a temporary escape from all

Early Diagnosis and Treatment Can Save Your Life

the madness, emotional drama, and pain by indulging in drugs. If anything takes you away from yourself and what you should be doing, it's toxic for you and needs to be left alone.

When my aunt died, I didn't go back home to her funeral. I had been to enough funerals in the past couple of years to last a lifetime. It seemed as if death was holding my hand. The family was on notice because we'd recently learned that my younger brother was very ill. My sisters, Barbara and Johnnie, had already gone back home to help my mother with Milton, who had been hospitalized. By the time we discovered the seriousness of his illness, he was in his final stages of full-blown AIDS. Six months later, he died.

While we knew my brother's death was inevitable, I don't think any of us expected it to come as quickly as it did. His funeral was the day before Mother's Day, which in itself was hard because I had to watch my mother mourn the loss of another son. (When my oldest brother died in Vietnam, I had to tell her the awful news; I was fifteen years old.) After Milton's funeral, it was hard leaving her. All of her children were scattered throughout the country and it meant one by one we would all have to return to our respective homes. She was left alone to grieve for her sister and her child. I prayed God would comfort her.

I arrived in Oakland on Monday, but did not immediately return to work because I'd caught a terrible cold while at home. Coupled with the stress of the funeral, I was thoroughly exhausted. Most of my co-workers and other department managers were very sympathetic. The Marketing/Membership department in which I worked was holding its usual Wednesday morning marketing meeting. When the meeting was over, my immediate supervisor called me into her office and fired me. Even though I was given prior approval, she said I'd taken too many days off for my brother's funeral. For just a brief moment I was stunned by my dismissal and wanted to lash out at her, but I quickly regained my composure. I knew she wanted a confrontation and I wouldn't give her the satisfaction. I thanked her for the opportunity of working with her and left. Life had given me enough drama and I wasn't up for any more.

I took the rest of the week off and started the following Monday looking for another job. I eventually landed a part-time position through a tem-

Early Diagnosis and Treatment Can Save Your Life

porary agency, working at Alameda County's Highland Hospital. I was on this assignment for approximately three weeks when I got the call from Peralta Community College District (PCCD) for a position there. While I liked my assignment at the hospital, I was looking forward to getting a full-time job with full-time benefits. Having medical coverage was important to me. I'd always had it and felt more secure with it.

Morning was not my best time of the day. At forty-two, I was already into my third year of menopause. Because I had such erratic sleeping habits, which accompanied all my other symptoms, it was difficult getting up. It took two alarm clocks to get me out of bed. The first clock was set for 6:00 a.m. to the sound of an alarm. I shut it off and turned over for the last thirty minutes of sleep, which was usually the best sleep. The second clock was set to alarm at 6:30 to music. Thank God for KBLX – The Quiet Storm. The morning DJ played the best jazz in the world.

With my eyes barely open, I rolled out of bed. One leg on the floor, lie there a few minutes, then the other, and lie a few more minutes. I mustered up enough energy and stumbled to the bathroom. I sat on the toilet for a few minutes collecting myself—stretching, scratching, moaning, and yawning. I finally got up and jumped in the shower. The water felt especially soothing, pulsating against my body, so I made the most of it and took an extra long shower. Since my interview wasn't until 9:00 o'clock, I had a lot of extra time that morning.

I emerged out of the shower feeling good, clean, and invigorated. I gently wiped the water off my face, ran the towel across my back, then gently patted the water off the right side of my body, starting at my breasts and working my way down. As I dried my left breast, I felt a lump on the underside of it. I wasn't even surprised by the lump.

"What's this?" I whispered to myself.

"I don't believe this. One of those bastards has bitten me again."

Our apartment was full of spiders. Two months prior, I awoke to discover a fairly good-sized lump on the same breast. I told George that a spider had bitten me. He wasn't so sure. We stripped down the bed, and sure enough, this creepy black and orange spider crawled from under my pillow.

Early Diagnosis and Treatment Can Save Your Life

The Diagnosis...My Journey Begins

I had almost convinced myself that this lump was just another spider bite, but it felt different. This lump was harder than the swollen, pus-filled one left by the spider. It also appeared to be within my breast instead of on top of my skin. I still didn't think there was cause for worry. So, I got dressed and was off to my interview.

After observing the lump for several more days, and being somewhat concerned because it hadn't gone down, I decided that I would have it checked out. I didn't have medical coverage, so I made an appointment at one of the clinics in the area that charged patients by their income. After a thorough clinical exam, the nurse practitioner ordered a mammogram and suggested I make the appointment as soon as possible. Breast cancer was never mentioned. I called the diagnostic center that was recommended by the nurse. My appointment was scheduled for the following week.

I didn't keep the appointment. I simply went about my regular routine, not having a care in the world. I did call to reschedule and was given another day to come in. I didn't tell anyone about my discovery. I don't even remember telling George right away. The lump just didn't seem that important or serious.

Nearly a month had passed since I discovered the lump. I was still working on temp assignments while I searched and interviewed for the perfect full-time job. In early June, I got the phone call from PCCD. I'd gotten the job that I had interviewed for earlier.

"When can you start?" Ms. Quinn asked.

"I can start right away, but I would like to give the hospital and the temp agency a two-week notice," I replied enthusiastically.

I was so excited about starting the new job that I missed my mammography appointment and had to reschedule it. I was very conscientious about not taking any days off during my ninety-day probationary period. Keeping the appointment didn't seem nearly as important as keeping a good job. I didn't keep the second appointment, or the third. And again, no one seemed particularly concerned that I had missed three scheduled mammography appointments. Not a phone call from the clinic, a letter, a call from the diagnostic center—nothing. So, I didn't feel there was any reason to be concerned. Besides, I was keeping an eye on the lump and there didn't appear to be any noticeable changes.

Early Diagnosis and Treatment Can Save Your Life

Finally, my ninety-day probationary period was over. It was now September and I had settled into my job as a full-time employee with benefits and medical coverage. One day while at work, I casually shared with my supervisor, Dena, that I'd discovered a lump. When I mentioned I'd found it months prior, she immediately became alarmed. This was the first time in four months that anyone had shown any concern the lump had not been examined.

Dena wasn't the typical supervisor to which I was accustomed. She was a very smart, dreadlock-wearing, tell-it-like-it-is sistah who cussed liked a drunken sailor. She had an unpretentious laugh, could be somewhat intimidating, but she had a generous heart, and could cook, act, and sing her butt off. We became good friends, and for the most part, she helped save my life.

"Girl, you better get your ass to the doctor," she demanded.

I made an appointment to have the mammography at Kaiser Permanente Hospital. Because I was a new patient, I had to be seen by a physician first. Normally, new patients would have to wait months to get an appointment with a doctor, but when I explained to the clerk that I had discovered the lump nearly four months prior; she found an opening for me immediately. (God works in mysterious ways, doesn't He? He placed me exactly where I needed to be.)

This was my first mammogram and I didn't know what to expect. The waiting area brimmed full of women - Caucasian, African American, Asian, young and old. While there, I ran into a friend. I found it odd that Tracey was having a mammography. She was only about twenty-six years old. She told me her breasts had been extremely sore and that she had felt a lump in her breast also. Her doctor recommended a mammogram, so she scheduled one right away. I told her about my discovery. We wished each other good luck as our names were called simultaneously.

I was ushered into a dormitory-type room with lockers, several benches, and small, enclosed dressing rooms. I was given a gown to put on. Once changed, I was directed to another waiting area until the technician came to get me.

The technician guided me to this machine that looked as if it was part robot and part gym apparatus. She asked me to remove the robe so

Early Diagnosis and Treatment Can Save Your Life

that my right breast could be x-rayed. She gently placed my breast between the two glass screens and began to compress the plates tightly.

"Hold your breath for a few seconds, please," she said as she stepped away to take the picture.

"Now, the left breast."

The technician followed the same procedure, taking several x-rays of both breasts. The pressing together of the two screens to hold the breasts wasn't as painful as it was uncomfortable. The entire process lasted less than twenty minutes.

When she was done, the young lady instructed me to have a seat in the waiting area. A short time later she and another more serious looking staff person approached me. The other person greeted me; I assumed this was the doctor. The technician stood there quietly. The doctor introduced herself.

"There are some suspicious images on the left breast and we need to take another set of pictures," the doctor said.

I was taken in for another set of x-rays. A short time later the two came out again. The doctor informed me that they wanted to schedule me for further testing. The ultrasound was scheduled for the following week. The first twinges of anxiety crept into my mind.

Unlike with my mammogram appointment, there was very little waiting time. I was quickly guided into a semi-dark examination room where I was immediately greeted by the technician. I was glad to see that the technician was a woman.

She spread the gel-like fluid on my left breast and began to maneuver the instrument over it. I watched the small monitor as she guided the hand-held instrument. Back and forth. Up and down. Special attention was given to the underside of my left breast. Within a few minutes the ultrasound was complete. The technician informed me that my doctor would discuss the results with me.

My concern about the seriousness of my condition was growing, as my appointment to see a doctor was a few days away. I arrived in the surgery department thirty minutes early and tried to remain calm. Within a short time, I was called into the examining room. Dr. June George entered shortly thereafter. She smiled as she entered and intro-

Early Diagnosis and Treatment Can Save Your Life

duced herself as she shook my hand. I instantly felt comfortable with her and liked her immediately. A soft-spoken woman with shoulder length, dark brown hair sprinkled with gray, she appeared to be in her mid-thirties.

She discussed the ultrasound results and told me she wanted to examine my breasts. I lay motionless on the table. As she performed the examination, she tried to reassure me but wanted me to know what the possible implications were. She seemed to genuinely care about my emotional well-being as well as my physical condition. I confided in her that I didn't see a doctor until nearly four months after I'd discovered the lump. I told her that no one seemed to be particularly concerned that I had missed numerous mammography appointments. I wasn't doctor bashing. I just wanted her to know I wasn't alarmed because no one else seemed to be. I realize now that my health care was my responsibility, not the doctor's.

"Well, let's see what's going on," she said somewhat cautiously.

Dr. George continued her examination. She informed me the ultrasound had shown not one, but two suspicious lumps on my left breast. And, to my shock, while she was examining me, she discovered what felt like another lump in my left armpit. Absolute fear and panic hit home. In a very compassionate voice, Dr. George told me she was going to perform a fine needle aspiration. She explained the procedure was being done to determine if the lumps were in fact benign cysts (just sacs of fluid) or something more serious.

She took out this large instrument with a needle on it that appeared to be three to four inches long. She wiped my breast with an antiseptic and gently inserted the needle into the first lump, which was located in the upper middle portion of my breast. When she withdrew the needle, there was blood in the syringe, no fluid. She placed the blood on a small piece glass and labeled it. Then she inserted the needle in the lump, which was located in the lower portion of my breast. And again, not much fluid came out, but it had more than the first lump. She labeled the specimen and said they would be sent to pathology immediately, with the results returning in a few days. My calm exterior belied my internal nervous breakdown.

Early Diagnosis and Treatment Can Save Your Life

A few days later, I received a call from Dr. George's office. Even though I didn't expect it so quickly, I was anxious to hear the results. I quickly left my office and made haste to the hospital. Once in the surgery department, I was immediately called and taken to an examination room. Dr. George entered shortly thereafter. We exchanged greetings and then she opened the chart she held in her hands.

"Some of the cells in the fluid appeared to be atypical," she said.

"What does that mean?" I questioned.

"Some of the cells appear to be abnormal and in order to determine the cause, I need to perform a biopsy."

"A biopsy?" I asked somewhat nervous.

"Yes, in order to take a closer look at the cells, I need to remove some of the tissue," Dr. George explained.

She scheduled the biopsy for the following week. For the first time since my discovery I was worried and fear started to take hold.

It was time to tell someone other than Dena. I told George first. Without giving too many details, I told him I had discovered a lump in my breast and the doctor needed to do some more tests. I finally found the courage to tell my daughter, Michelle, that I had to go have a biopsy performed. I didn't mention the words "breast cancer" because I didn't want to upset her unnecessarily. Nor did I allow myself to think that I could possibly have any disease, let alone cancer.

George and I had been seeing each other on and off for nearly ten years. At the time of my diagnosis, we weren't together as a couple, but we maintained a very good friendship and shared a house together. I knew that George would be there for me and my family would be supportive as well, but this was one of those times that I needed my best friend.

I wished Jo could have been here to help me get through this. I could tell her what I was feeling and share my secret fears with her. I needed my best friend to lean on. She would know the right things to say and the right things to do. She would make sure that I was taken care of, that I was safe. I missed her terribly and it was as if I was going through the grieving process all over again.

I kept the pre-surgery screening appointment as scheduled. The

Early Diagnosis and Treatment Can Save Your Life

scheduling nurse gave me a list of instructions; complete with a map of where I should go when I arrived at the hospital. After making sure she had all the patient information in terms of my medical history, allergies, next of kin, who would bring me and pick me up from the hospital, etc., she gave me a pamphlet about breast cancer. She told me that she didn't want to alarm me, but that she was required by law to give me the information. She also told me I probably shouldn't read it until after I got the biopsy results. I left the doctor's office, went home, stuck the pamphlet in my drawer and didn't think about it again. My biopsy was scheduled for the next day.

I followed the pre-surgery instructions to the letter. The night before the surgery I could not eat or drink anything, not even water. I was told not to put on any lotion, perfume, or deodorant. I had some problems with the instructions, but I knew I had to follow them.

I said another prayer before I left home. The early morning ride to the hospital was quiet. George and I talked very little. He sat in the waiting area until my name was called. We stood simultaneously and gave each other a hug.

"I'll see you later, Nikki," he said, somewhat worried.

The nurse and I rode the elevator in silence. I was directed to an area where I changed into the standard hospital gear. I was then escorted to another room, placed on a gurney and wheeled into a large operating room. The room, bright and full of instruments, was very, very cold. I gladly accepted the extra blanket the nurse offered. I was told during my pre-surgery consultation I would be given just enough anesthesia to relax me, but I would be aware of what was going on and could communicate with the doctors. I'd always thought you had to be completely out during surgery so I was fascinated by this new procedure.

The medical team entered the operating room. One of nurses inserted the intravenous needle in my right hand. The anesthesiologists stood just behind my head and begin to administer the sedative. I could feel myself becoming lightheaded, my body completely relaxing.

"Good morning, Nicole, how are you?" Dr. George asked as she entered the room.

"I'm okay, I think."

Early Diagnosis and Treatment Can Save Your Life

The Diagnosis...My Journey Begins

"Do you know what we're going to be doing today?" Dr. George asked.

"Yes, you're going to remove some tissue from my left breast, at least that's what you told me you were going to do."

Some of the staff laughed.

"Correct," she said in her soft-spoken voice.

Dr. George began the procedure by making a small incision on the upper part of my breast. As she made the incision, I could feel the pressure of the knife moving across my chest. I told Dr. George that I could feel the scalpel. She instructed the anesthesiologist to give me a little more sedative and then she proceeded. Another incision was made on the underside of my breast. When all the tissue had been removed, I asked Dr. George if I could see it.

"Are you sure, Nicole?" she questioned.

A portion of tissue was placed in a small, stainless steel dish and one of the nurses brought it over to me. I was amazed to see the mass of tissue looked like the yellowish fat that is found on chicken, except that it was thicker and had tiny blood vessels on it.

The entire procedure took less than an hour. The incisions were sutured and I was moved to recovery. There were no complications, so my stay in the recovery room was short. I was given some pain medication along with post-op directions, which instructed me not to drive a car, operate mechanical equipment or make important decisions for at least twenty-four hours. George picked me up and after only a few hours of rest, I was back to normal. I felt well enough to return to work the next day.

On Friday of the following week, I received the phone call from Dr. George's office.

"Ms. Bryant, the results of the biopsy are in and Dr. George would like to see you as soon as possible."

I hesitated briefly, and then told her I would be there shortly.

I told Dena I had to leave work because the doctor's office called. I then phoned George to tell him the results were in and asked if he could meet me at the hospital after he picked Briannah up from school.

I decided to take the bus to the hospital because it was more conven-

Early Diagnosis and Treatment Can Save Your Life

ient and the ride from my job took less than fifteen minutes. That is, any other time it would have. But not this ride. It seemed as if I rode for hours. It was no doubt the longest ride of my life. Fear set in as I agonized about the impending results. I kept telling myself I had to remain optimistic. I knew that getting the results was important, but I was so afraid of the outcome that I didn't want to know.

I pulled out the newspaper I had purchased while waiting on the bus and began to read. The very first article on the front page of the newspaper immediately caught my attention. The caption read "Local Hospital Receives New Magnetic Imaging Machine." The first two sentences of the article contained two words that I had become familiar with—mammogram and breast cancer. I immediately closed the newspaper and laid it down in the empty seat next to me. I rode the rest of the way just sitting, trying not to think, oblivious to all the activity on the bus.

I finally arrived at the surgery department waiting area. I sat in the chair and picked up a magazine. To my surprise, the heading on the front cover read "National Breast Cancer Awareness Month." I had never heard of a month being designated for breast cancer awareness. I reluctantly flipped a few pages of the magazine and put it down. I knew in my heart these were two more signs of bad news. Earlier that morning while I was getting dressed, the morning news aired a segment on breast cancer. I didn't really pay much attention to what was being said because I was getting ready for work. In retrospect, I rationalized that all these signs were omens of bad things to come.

George and Briannah walked into the waiting area. I tried to put on a brave face, but I'm sure George could tell I was worried.

"Hi NaNa," Briannah said as she ran over to greet me.

"You all right?" he asked.

"Yeah, I think so."

I was anything but all right. I was scared. The nurse called my name and I followed her past the reception area and into an examining room. When Dr. George entered the room I was sitting on the examining table. I couldn't tell from her facial expression if the news was good or bad, but when she starting talking, the tone of her voice wasn't what I had been

Early Diagnosis and Treatment Can Save Your Life

accustomed to hearing. A hint of sadness penetrated her typically soft tone.

"Hello, Nicole. How are you holding up?"

"Pretty good, I guess." By now, I had become pretty good at pretending.

"Nicole, I have good news and bad news, which do you want first?" she asked solemnly.

"The bad news first," I said somewhat jokingly. "That way the last thing I hear will be something good."

I knew this was no joking matter.

Dr. George took a small breath.

"The lump that was located in the upper portion of your breast was malignant; it's cancer."

I took a deep breath. The room went completely black, like someone was holding a cloak over my head. Nothing but darkness existed. No sounds of any kind. I'd heard enough about that word "malignant" to know that it wasn't good. "Malignant" hung in mid-air like a feather slowly circling the room and descending into the darkness. I saw death. I fought to hold back the tears but couldn't.

"Oh God, please please no," I cried. "Don't let this happen to me. Please God, no. Please let the test be wrong," I silently begged.

Dr. George stood there patiently, waiting for me to get that first cry out. I managed to compose myself long enough to hear Dr. George ask me if I was okay. Finally, for the first time in months I didn't have to pretend.

"No, I am not okay," I replied, barely able to get the words out.

"What's the good news?" I asked pitifully.

Dr. George proceeded to explain that the lump located in the lower part of my breast was benign and that the lumps under my arm were just fatty tissue.

I was now crying uncontrollably. While I was glad to hear the 'good' news, I was totally devastated by the 'bad' news. Dr. George asked if I had someone with me. Even though I heard her, it was as if her mouth was moving but no words were coming out. I was still trying to digest the fact I had cancer. I don't think I heard much else of what she said. Everything from that point on was in super slow motion,

Early Diagnosis and Treatment Can Save Your Life

almost inaudible. I completely shut down. I didn't want to hear any more of what she had to say. I think, no I'm sure, I briefly left my body. My body was still sitting on the examining table, but my spirit was someplace else. It wasn't me being told that I had cancer. It couldn't be me. Surely, the diagnosis was wrong. I wasn't sick, and I certainly didn't have breast cancer. I didn't feel sick, I didn't look sick. It had to be a mistake.

"Is there a chance the results were wrong?" I asked in an almost childlike voice.

"No, we're certain that the results were correct," she replied.

My mind was racing.

"Dr. George, how did I get this?" I asked crying through my words.

"No one knows where it comes from, Nicole; we just don't know. I know it's a lot for you to take in. I know it's scary for you right now and I do understand your fear."

I covered my face with my hands. I couldn't stop crying. My heart was pounding; my head hurt, my body was limp. I just wanted to go home. At that moment, I just wanted to lie down and sleep into death.

Dr. George began to explain what I needed to do next and discussed my treatment options.

"There are several courses of action we can take."

I was glad to hear her say "we" because I didn't have a clue what to do. She took out a pink piece of paper, drew five horizontal lines across it. I watched, silently crying, as she began writing.

— Mastectomy (removes breast and lymph nodes) – possible chemotherapy, possible radiation therapy.
— Lumpectomy and lymph node dissection – definite radiation therapy (six weeks); possible chemotherapy.
— May be recommended to have chemo first.
— Surgeon
— Oncologist
— Radiation Oncologist
— Breast Care Coordinator
— American Cancer Society/Reach to Recovery

Early Diagnosis and Treatment Can Save Your Life

As she continued to write the information, Dr. George would stop occasionally to ask me if I was okay. In the last section, she also wrote her office number, her personal pager number, and her hospital pager number, along with the name of the Breast Care Coordinator, Lynette Beckley. She recommended I make an appointment to see Ms. Beckley as soon possible.

I sat on the table, unable to move. Dr. George began to speak again.

"I realize that this has been a lot to digest. However, I want you to start thinking seriously about your treatment options. You have an aggressive cancer, but it's one of the most common forms of breast cancer. I encourage you to get a second opinion if that will ease your mind. As a matter of fact, I would prefer you do so. If you decide you want to get a second opinion, it is important you contact a physician right away. I want to give you some time, but I would like to start your surgery within the next thirty days. Let me know what you decide to do. I know it's a lot for you to do in a short period of time. But the sooner we get started, the better."

Dr. George ended the session and suggested that I take the rest of the day off from work.

"Do you have someone here with you, Nicole?"

"Yes, my friend and granddaughter are here with me, but I need to call my job."

"You can use the phone in my office," she replied.

I slowly slid off the examining table and followed Dr. George to her office. I sat in the chair at her desk for a few moments before I dialed the number. The phone rang several times and Dena answered. The moment I heard her voice I began to cry a little bit. I was barely able to say the words.

"Dena, the lump was breast cancer."

"No, Nicole," Dena sighed, clearly shaken.

Neither one of us said anything else for a few seconds. I finally told her I was going to go home and I would see her Monday morning. After hanging up the phone, I sat in the chair for a few moments. With my arms folded on the desk, I placed my head on them and cried. The darkness that appeared in the examining room now cast its shadow as I sat

Early Diagnosis and Treatment Can Save Your Life

in Dr. George's office. The first thought that came to my mind was I would not be around to see my granddaughters grow up.

"Oh God, please help me; don't let me die," I silently pleaded.

I composed myself and walked back to the waiting area. I saw George and Briannah before they saw me. As soon as Briannah saw me, she ran over to me. George immediately stood up. Right away, he knew something was wrong. I didn't want Briannah to see me cry or see how upset I was, so I gave her a hug without really looking her in the face. Only five years old at the time, I knew I could fool her—but not George. I turned to him and without saying a word, I nodded my head yes. He took Briannah's and my hand as we walked out the hospital.

Early Diagnosis and Treatment Can Save Your Life

> *Everything in our lives happens for a reason. We may not understand or know the reason why, but it is according to God's plan and His purpose.*
>
> **Lessons from my life's journey**

3
Devastated But Not Destroyed

On the ride home, I made small talk with Briannah about school. Aside from that, I didn't say much. Briannah was always talkative, but she was particularly a chatterbox that day. Wouldn't you know it, on the day I received the worst news of my life, my baby wanted to tell me everything she'd done in kindergarten that day. For the first time in her little life, I wished she would shut up. I sat quietly as she went on and on about her day at school, and this little boy who was always hitting her, and that she wanted some shrimp fried rice. She was driving me crazy.

Finally, I was home. I could shut down from the world. I didn't want to see anyone, talk to anyone, or do anything. I just wanted to lie down. I dragged myself up the stairs and went straight to my bedroom. I sat on the side of the bed numb in disbelief, fractured to what I thought was beyond repair. I was devastated. Most of all, I was scared; almost too afraid to draw another breath for fear it would be my last.

George entered the bedroom and sat next to me. Neither one of us knew what to say to each other. He gave me a reassuring pat on my thigh as if to say everything would be okay. We had an unusual relationship. At the time of my diagnosis, it was during one of our "off" periods. While we lived together and even slept in the same bed, we weren't intimate. I think at the time we both were going through some type of mid-life crisis. In spite of our unorthodox arrangement, it worked for us. I could call on him for anything. And likewise, I would do the same for him. My family liked him, and my granddaughters, especially Briannah, absolutely adored him. He certainly was a good man and an even better friend.

George allowed me some time to myself. As I lay across the bed, I couldn't rest because my mind was racing. I knew Michelle would be coming home soon. How in the world was I going to tell her? My tears briefly lulled me to sleep. When I awoke, I heard George and Briannah going to the door. It was Michelle and her friend, Shelly.

"Hi, Mom," Michelle called out.

Early Diagnosis and Treatment Can Save Your Life

No sooner had I sat on the bed she entered my room. Shelly was few steps behind her.

"What did the doctor say?" she asked anxiously.

I wasn't prepared to tell her so soon after hearing it myself.

How do you tell someone you love that you have cancer and that you could possibly die?

Just as it had been with George, when I looked in her eyes, she knew.

So I just said it.

"The doctor said that it was breast cancer."

"Are they sure, Mom?"

"That's what the test showed and the doctor said the tumor was malignant," I replied.

"Wow, Mom," she said softly, as she walked over to me and gave me a hug.

On the surface, Michelle took the news better than I expected, but I could see she was upset. Even she couldn't hide the sadness in those big eyes as they ballooned with tears. I really think she was trying to be strong for me.

"Are you okay, Ms. Nikki?" Shelly asked.

"Yeah, I'm okay."

"Did your doctor give you something to calm your nerves?" Shelly inquired.

"No, I don't need anything," I replied.

"Well, I think she should have given you something. I'm going to go home and get some of my grandmother's Valium for you. They will help you calm your nerves so that you can rest."

Before I could even respond, Shelly and Michelle were out the door.

They returned just as quickly as they had left. I was still in the exact same spot on my bed—my body frozen, my thoughts rapidly engaged. I imagined these Ms. Pac Man type creatures growing, as one consumed the other until my body was ravaged. I envisioned my own funeral. Maybe I did need something to relax me. Shelly put the Valium on the nightstand.

Michelle asked me again if I was going to be all right. I told her that

Early Diagnosis and Treatment Can Save Your Life

I would. While I appreciated their concern, I really wanted to be left alone. I asked both of them not to say anything to the family yet. I wanted to tell them myself, in my own way and time. She gave me another hug then they made their way to the door. I could hear the front door open. Then Michelle came back into my bedroom.

"What about JuJu?" Michelle asked.

"You can tell him if you want," I mumbled.

I agreed to let her tell her brother because I knew she probably couldn't keep something like that to herself, and especially from him. I don't know if it would have even been fair to ask her not to tell him.

JuJu called later that night. Like George and Michelle, I don't think he knew what to say. He seemed to handle the news okay, considering. I wasn't much up to talking so I told him I was exhausted and wanted to rest. I wasn't tired as much as I just didn't want to talk about it anymore. The realization of having cancer hadn't sunk in yet. I needed time to process the fact that I had it. I needed time to accept the fact that my life was no longer mine.

This was something new for all of us. While we'd had tragedies in our family, this was the first time that our strength as an immediate unit (mother, son, and daughter) had been tested. I didn't want to think about anything else for the rest of the night. Knowing that my children knew somehow made it worse for me. I anguished about what they might be going through. So I took Shelly's advice and took the Valium. I took two of the pills and put the remainder on my nightstand.

I laid across the bed, almost lifeless, for a couple of hours. I don't know if it was from the Valium or from sheer emotional exhaustion. It didn't really matter at that point. Later that night I asked George if he would go to the store and get me something to drink. I figured some wine wouldn't hurt. Besides, I already had cancer. Pills, booze, drugs, nothing was going to do any more damage than the cancer would. He brought me back a bottle of wine. In addition to the wine and pills, I also consumed some cocaine. In retrospect, I don't know what I was thinking. But, at that moment, I didn't care; I didn't want to feel life. The enormity of having this disease was too much for me.

Even in my pill-induced, drug and alcohol state, I prayed that God

Early Diagnosis and Treatment Can Save Your Life

watched over me. I continued this destructive behavior all night Friday, all day Saturday and most of Saturday night. I'm not sure what time it was when I finally went to sleep Saturday night, but I woke up around 5:00 a.m. that Sunday morning to use the bathroom. While sitting on the toilet, I began to cry. This cry was different from all the previous episodes; my soul spoke. I sat there and silently prayed. I wanted help, I needed help, and I knew that I couldn't do it alone. I also knew that I didn't want this disease to destroy me.

"Oh God, please help me. Dear God in Heaven, please don't leave now. You have watched over me and protected me all my life. You have stuck by me and comforted me. I know lately I haven't acted much like your child. But I am your child and you know that I need you right now more than I ever have. I'm asking you to please help me and to heal me. I'm sick, I'm scared, and I don't know what to do, but I know you do. Anoint me with your healing hands. I love you Lord and I know you love me. Please help me. Give me the strength to fight this disease, please heal me. Let your perfect will be done. These things I ask in your son Jesus' name, Amen."

I quietly crawled back into bed. I knew that God heard my prayers, but I wasn't sure if He would answer them. Lately, I hadn't been acting like I knew Him, so I couldn't blame Him if he rejected me. My mother always used to say that God might not come when you want Him, but He's always there when you need Him and He always comes on time. I was relying on this and on His Word that He loved me. No matter what, He would answer the prayers of all his children, saints and sinners alike.

When I awoke later that morning, I was ready to do whatever I needed in order to live. First, I had to learn about this disease. I took out all the literature on breast cancer the nurse had given me during my pre-surgery consultation. I scoured through the papers in my purse and found the name and phone number of Gillie, a friend of Dena's. Gillie, who lived in Washington, D.C., was a breast cancer survivor. We'd only talked once shortly after my biopsy. I didn't know anyone else who was a breast cancer survivor, so Gillie was it, and I was eager to learn about this disease.

The phone rang numerous times. I was afraid that since it was Sunday and because of our time difference she might be at church. Relief came when I heard her voice. We talked for quite a while. She provided me

Early Diagnosis and Treatment Can Save Your Life

with enough information so that I would at least know what to do and to expect. But more than anything, she gave me hope. She was a survivor! Gillie had been diagnosed with a rare form of breast cancer and was nearing her five-year anniversary. She made me realize that my survival was based on several things: the stage of my cancer, my willingness to do all I could do to fight and God's will.

Even though I'd accepted my diagnosis and made my decision to fight, that little voice of self-doubt remained. I lingered in a scary place. Wanting to live, unsure of my future, but scared to death of what lay ahead. I still had a lot to do. First, I had to tell the rest of my family, close friends, then Nathan, whom I had recently started dating.

I had seven sisters. Because I had a different relationship with each one of them and each had a very unique personality, my initial thought was to tell them individually. The more I thought about it, the more I realized that I didn't want to have to repeat it seven times. Luckily, I didn't have to torture myself. I started calling them late Sunday evening. By the time I told one, another sister was calling me saying she had heard the news. Each handled it differently and each gave me words of encouragement. While I'm sure they, like me, were devastated by the news, each one of them tried to be positive. All of them were very concerned about how I was doing.

Of all their responses, Barbara's was the most memorable.

"Girl, don't worry about it. You'll be okay. It's just a titty. He can't suck but one titty at a time anyway. Besides, you can still f. . . , can't you?"

You had to know Barbara and understand her personality to appreciate her sense of humor and response.

"Yeah, you have a good point," I replied, when I finally stopped laughing.

My biggest concern was telling my mother (whom we called Lil' Mama). I didn't want her worrying about losing another child while she was still mourning the loss of my brother. It had only been five months since his death. I figured once I got past telling her, everyone else would be easy. I waited a few days before I finally got the courage to call. Much to my surprise and relief, one of my sisters had already told her. I reassured her I would be okay and that she shouldn't worry about me.

"Listen to your Lil' Mama," she said in a reassuring voice.

Early Diagnosis and Treatment Can Save Your Life

"God won't put no more on you than you can bear. Just keep on praying and asking Him to heal you."

"I know, Lil' Mama."

Lil' Mama was a strong woman whose faith was steadfast and believed in the power of prayer. She lived by that adage. I heard her say it so many times when I was growing up. With each crisis she faced, she appeared to get stronger. I often wondered how she did it. I suppose in some ways I was a beneficiary of that strength. I just didn't know it yet.

Dr. George made an appointment for me to see the Breast Care Coordinator at Kaiser. I arrived somewhat emotionally drained but knew seeing her was part of the process. Ms. Beckley gave me a lot of literature, most of which was overwhelming. It did, however, give me some idea of the challenges that awaited me. She asked if she could contact the American Cancer Society on my behalf and gave me the names of several other organizations and support groups that I might be interested in calling.

Aside from possibly dying from this disease, my biggest fear was how my body would look if I opted for the mastectomy. I was leaning towards it as a treatment option. I'd never seen a picture of anyone who had a mastectomy. I envisioned this grotesque chittlin-like crater being left where my breast once was. Ms. Beckley told me if I had had surgery more than ten years ago that's exactly what my chest would have looked like. This wasn't very comforting. I asked her if she had a picture of a woman with a mastectomy, hoping it would be of an African American female.

When she showed me a picture of an older white woman, I cried. According to Ms. Beckley, the woman in the picture received her mastectomy at least ten years prior to my diagnosis. The picture wasn't very flattering. Not that any picture of a woman whose breast had been removed would have been, but I just needed to see someone with whom I could relate. Certainly there were other African American women who had had a mastectomy. All of my anxieties and fears returned. Maybe a mastectomy wasn't the best choice. I was more convinced than ever that I needed to get a second opinion.

As soon as I returned to work, I got busy calling around for recom-

Early Diagnosis and Treatment Can Save Your Life

mendations of a doctor who could give me a second opinion. Then I remembered an article I'd read about Alta Bates Hospital Comprehensive Breast Center. I called the hospital and was given an appointment to speak to the Breast Center's Second Opinion Consultation Team. I received confirmation in the mail stating that my appointment was scheduled for Wednesday, October 19th from 1:30 to 5:30 p.m. The letter was very formal and offered words that certainly made me more at ease about seeing them: *This service makes available to you some of the Bay Area's most knowledgeable cancer experts for a full second opinion review of your breast cancer diagnosis. In addition to reviewing your diagnosis, our physicians will also review key tests performed to assess the extent of the breast cancer, conduct a physical examination, and issue treatment recommendations to your primary care or other designated physician.*

The team comprised a dozen members, including a medical oncologist, surgeon, radiation oncologist, pathologist, radiologist, plastic surgeon, psychiatrist, psycho-socialist, program director, nurse coordinator, the program chair, and a physician who specialized in cancer risk counseling. Prior to my appointment, I had to send my most recent pathology report, recent mammogram screenings, copies of my medical records, and lab tests, along with other relevant reports and recommendations.

I was cautiously optimistic about being seen by this team of experts; hoping they would give me a different diagnosis. At the same time, I was somewhat terrified by the thought that this team could find a more serious diagnosis than that of Dr. George's. In any event, I was certain that after the session I would be better equipped to make a rational and realistic decision about my treatment option. I prayed the diagnosis would be different.

My consultation lasted almost five hours. The services included a clinical breast exam, instructions on how to perform a self-breast exam, and a session with the social worker. I met with several other specialists and finally I met with the team chair to discuss the panel's recommendations. As it turned out, their diagnosis matched that of Dr. George's. One of the physicians even suggested that I consider a lumpectomy as a

Early Diagnosis and Treatment Can Save Your Life

treatment option. I had to make a decision and decide within a reasonably short period of time.

The team of physicians gave me more information about breast cancer. While most of it was pretty much the same, I still learned some new things. I returned to work the next day and immediately became a breast cancer sleuth. I went on the Internet, to the library, and called the other hospitals in the area to see what information they had. I also received a lot of information from Kaiser Hospital's education center. A co-worker recommended several books to read that would help prepare me for surgery, both physically and emotionally. I immersed myself in so much information I barely had time for anything else.

Even though all the literature I read stated otherwise, I couldn't help but wonder if I had done something that caused me to get this disease. Could I have done something, anything, which would have prevented me from getting cancer? I convinced myself that I had done something at some point in my life that caused this because none of the women in my immediate family had the disease. There was a nation of women in my family, and to my knowledge, not one of them had been diagnosed with breast cancer, any cancer for that matter.

I thought back to when I was a kid growing up in East Carondelet. For the most part, we ate really well. My mother and grandmother grew their vegetables. I didn't have my first McDonald's burger until I was nearly sixteen, so fast food wasn't a big part of my diet. Could it have been caused from the chemicals that were sprayed in our neighborhood during the summer months? We would run and play through the thick plume of smoke trailing the pesticide truck that sprayed for mosquitoes. Could it have come from the toxic vapor clouds released from the chemical plant that was in the area?

Having ruled out things in my childhood, I concentrated on potential causes from my adulthood. Maybe it was from the fumes coming through the exhaust into my car? I drove my car for at least ten years with that problem. Could it have come from all the stress I had gone through during the previous years? Maybe it came from the polluted environment—the air we breathe, the water we drink, the food we eat—it's all contaminated to some degree. I was making myself crazy. The

Early Diagnosis and Treatment Can Save Your Life

answers to my questions weren't in the literature I was reading. Consequently, I could not hold myself blameless for being in this predicament.

To some degree, I had accepted the diagnosis, but feelings of sadness and despair seem to always return. I was glad we would soon be setting the surgery date; I wanted to rid my body of this deadly invader. But on the other hand, I was scared everything would be different. If I survived the operation, could I survive the disease? Could I survive unlearning all society had taught me about body image and beauty? There was still so much I didn't know about breast cancer. I would be faced with new limitations, new restrictions, and new challenges. My fears about my own mortality coupled with worrying about not being around to see my granddaughters grow up, to give them advice and to protect them, were overwhelming.

I met with Dr. George a few days after seeing the physicians at Alta Bates. As always, she was pleasant and very easy to talk to. I shared with her the information from the medical team and told her they concurred with her diagnosis. They did, however, suggest that I consider the lumpectomy as a treatment option. Dr. George had additional lab results as well. She provided me with more information about the type and stage of my cancer. My avocado seed-size tumor was typed as Stage II Infiltrating Ductile Carcinoma. Its technical name made it seem even more ominous.

We discussed my treatment options, lumpectomy or mastectomy. If I decided on the lumpectomy, I would **have** to be subjected to a series of chemotherapy and radiation treatments. If I chose the mastectomy, it would mean that my entire breast would be removed. Chemotherapy and radiation would depend on whether the cancer had metastasized, if there was lymph node involvement, or used as a possible preventive measure. I didn't like the idea of having months of chemotherapy and radiation treatments on top of a disfigured breast. Nor was I totally thrilled with having my breast amputated. My choices were few, but I was very certain that I didn't want to subject myself to any more pain and suffering than absolutely necessary. I wasn't particularly thrilled about either choice. Each had its advantages and disadvantages, but I had to choose one.

Early Diagnosis and Treatment Can Save Your Life

"What would you do, Dr. George?" I asked her.

"I can't answer that, Nicole," she replied. "You'll have to make your decision based on what you feel is best for you."

I suppose I was trying to get out of taking responsibility for making a decision I would regret later. Dr. George, and rightly so, would not allow me to relinquish that responsibility. The hardest part was making the decision. Once I made it, I was relieved. Both choices were bad, so I chose what I thought was the lesser of the two evils. More than anything, I chose the one I thought would give me a better chance at surviving this monster. I decided to have the mastectomy. The date was set: Saturday, October 29, 1994.

During the course of the next few days, almost everyone that mattered to me had been told—my family, my two closest friends, Heather and Marsha, some extended family members, and a few co-workers. I still hadn't told Nathan. I put it off because I didn't know what to say, how to say it or the right time to tell him.

I'd met Nathan just after I started working at Laney College. His Alameda County Transit bus route took him right past my job. On those days when I didn't feel like walking home, I would ride the bus. After several months of talking, there was clearly an attraction. We shared an interest in football and spent hours over the phone talking about our lives, relationships, and sports. During one of our conversations, he revealed to me that he was a "breast and leg man." Knowing that information and our relationship being relatively new, I didn't know if it would survive once I lost a breast. Consequently, I avoided the subject.

It would have been nice if there had been a manual to instruct me step by step on when to tell him, where to tell, and what to say to him. I just didn't know how. In all the information I read, and there was a lot, none of the articles dealt with the impact of breast cancer on your relationship, intimacy, body image, and sex after breast cancer. I was too busy trying to learn about the disease and how to keep myself healthy rather than learning how to cope afterwards. I hadn't even considered how he would handle this. I decided to put off telling him until I was sure what I was going to do in terms of my treatment options. That was

Early Diagnosis and Treatment Can Save Your Life

my rationalization; however, I knew I eventually would have to tell him. I wasn't comfortable with the disease; how could I expect him to be?

I phoned Nathan and told him that I had something important to tell him. While he knew I had being seeing several doctors, I didn't share with him why. I just told him I was having some tests done. He picked me up and we went to our favorite spot at the Berkeley Marina. Nathan always greeted me with the biggest smile. He had perfect white teeth, the warmest smile, and the sexiest, Barry White-sounding voice. We sat at a small table in a corner of the restaurant that facing the water. He ordered two glasses of wine. We made small talk, sharing the events of the day, talked a bit about football. I took another sip of wine and then in a whisper, said it.

"Nathan, I have breast cancer and I've decided to have my breast removed."

He appeared somewhat shaken by the news. The big smile disappeared; worry took its place.

"Wow, when did all this happen? Are you sure?" he asked.

"Yes, I'm sure, and I've known a little over month. I'm scheduled to have surgery in a few weeks."

"A few weeks?" he responded, almost in disbelief.

It had become a familiar pattern. Like everyone else, he too was searching for the right words to say. The once-happy, strong man was gone. The eyes of a sad little boy surfaced. His reaction made me return the same emotion. I didn't know what his reaction would be, but I didn't expect him to be so affected by it. Even though this was a serious matter, I knew I needed to do or say something to lighten things up.

"Well, it could be worse you know. It could have been one of my legs," I said jokingly.

He recovered with a quick little smile.

"Girl, not the leg, anything but one of those fine legs of yours."

I took his hand into mine, leaned over and gently kissed him on his lips.

"See, when you think about it, it's not so bad after all, huh? We'll just have to get more creative, won't we?" I said flirtatiously.

A glimpse of a smile reappeared. The conversation turned serious again.

"I don't want you to worry about me because I'm going to be just fine. I've got an excellent doctor and my hospital stay will only be for

Early Diagnosis and Treatment Can Save Your Life

a few days."

"Why didn't you tell me earlier?"

"I couldn't bring myself to tell you."

There was a long period of silence. For the first time since we'd starting dating, I felt strangely awkward, out of place, and speechless. I could see that he was just as uncomfortable talking about the cancer and my surgery as I was, so I quickly changed the subject back to football. This was something we both enjoyed talking about.

We finished our drinks and left the bar. During the drive home, we both were pretty quiet. We took the Frontage Road along the Berkeley Marina. I asked Nathan to stop for a minute. He pulled off the side of the road. I rolled the window down. It was so dark outside that I couldn't see where the water ended and the shore began. In the distance, the lights from San Francisco were visible. "If I Could" by Regina Bell was playing on the radio. We sat there quietly listening to Regina belt out her tune…

"If I could I would protect you from the sadness that's in your eyes; give you courage in a world of compromise. If I could in a time and place where you don't want to be...But I would, if I could."

It was as if the DJ knew my situation and was playing songs that would soothe my soul—Frankie Beverly & Maze, Luther, the Whispers, Smokey's "Quiet Storm." One minute we were listening to the music, quietly sitting in the darkness, watching the moonlight. The next moment, we were kissing passionately, and then making love.

I don't even know how we managed, given the very small space in the truck. Nathan was a little over six feet. I'd always been somewhat spontaneous and uninhibited, but even for me, this was a bit much. At the time, getting caught, not to mention arrested, didn't matter. Of course afterwards, we both realized how careless we had been. But neither one of us was going to beat ourselves up about it. Maybe there's some truth to what they say about when you think you're going to die you take more chances with life. Nathan managed to drive all the way to my house with one arm around me and the other on the steering wheel. It was nice.

The closer it got to the surgery date, the more the realization I had breast cancer crystallized. I accepted I had the disease, and managed to

Early Diagnosis and Treatment Can Save Your Life

put up a good front. I'd done all the things that I could do physically to prepare myself for the surgery. I walked daily, took my vitamins, got plenty of rest, and watched my eating habits. I went through the physical mechanics, but I realized there was so much more to do. I hadn't prepared myself for the emotional fallout. I wasn't even sure what the fallout would be. Uncertain and vulnerable, the only thing I could do was pray and wait to see what would come.

Early Diagnosis and Treatment Can Save Your Life

> *Be merciful unto me, O God; be merciful unto me for my soul trusteth in Thee: Yea, in the shadow of thy wings I will make my refuge, until these calamities be over past.*
>
> **Psalm 57:1**

4

The Emancipation of My Symbol of Beauty

It had been nearly a month since I learned breast cancer had invaded my body. I was relieved the surgery was going to take place relatively soon. I made sure everything I had to do was done. I prepared my list of "things to do" before going into the hospital. I checked them off as I completed each task. I let Michelle know where all my important papers were, just in case. All the bills had been paid. All the papers for the surgery were in order. There was enough food in the house for Michelle and Briannah. I bought a new gown and slippers, packed my suitcase full of my favorite toiletries and lotions. One would have thought I was going away for a month. My entire stay in the hospital was estimated to be a few days at the most. My last "to do" was to get my hair braided. I was told that I might not be able to lift my arm over my head for a while. It's amazing how cancer complicates the simplest of tasks.

I began to second-guess my decision to have the surgery. I still had questions, and a lot of doubt. I foolishly wondered if I even had breast cancer at all. Maybe I should get a third opinion, I thought to myself. I knew deep down the diagnosis would be the same even if I'd gone to see 100 doctors. I was just scared. Scared the cancer had gotten worse since the biopsy, halfway believing in those myths about the disease spreading once you've been cut, and uncertain if I would be able to live with my decision to have my breast removed. When I was first diagnosed, I was scared to death of dying and confused about whether I wanted to live. Even though I read articles about the survival rates, I didn't find much comfort in them—African American women were dying at alarming rates. As a result, I wasn't convinced of my chances of surviving.

Attending church had not been on my list of priorities over the years, but I did have the good sense to pray on a regular basis. I felt almost guilty about asking God to help me. I hadn't given Him much time in the past years. Consequently, I was on an emotional and spiritual roller coaster. Some days I was really confident and optimistic about my

Early Diagnosis and Treatment Can Save Your Life

future; my faith was strong. Other days I was sad, like a scared little girl, apprehensive about everything. Interestingly enough, I didn't let anyone around me know how I was feeling. I especially didn't want my children to know just how frightened and emotionally fragile I was. I wanted them to believe that I was going to be okay. It was important for me to project that.

There was a time when I actually considered taking my own life. Shortly after the diagnosis I was walking to work when I thought to myself: *I could just stop right here in the middle of this street and it would all be over. I wouldn't have to worry about breast cancer, chemotherapy or anything. I could end my life right now, right here.* On another occasion, I thought about ending my life by taking the bottle of pain pills the doctor had given me. I knew in my heart that I didn't want to die, nor would I do anything to harm myself, but Satan has a way of getting really busy when you are weak and in despair. I knew ending my life went against everything I had been taught about God, prayer, and faith. I knew my faith was being tested like it never had been before. My will to live was stronger than my fear of the cancer.

The closer it got to the surgery date, the more I thought about not having the operation. That Thursday prior to the surgery, I was at the bank conducting some business. One of my friends was a teller at the bank and we were discussing my surgery. She told me she would pray for me. As I exited, a woman who was standing behind me in the line approached me. She suggested I might want to reconsider having such invasive surgery and I should look into alternative treatments. She encouraged me to try a holistic approach by taking vitamins and herbs to shrink the tumor. A friend of hers had been successfully cured of breast cancer without surgery. She even gave me a card with the name of the holistic doctor she recommended I use.

While I had read a little bit about alternative medicines in treating breast cancer, I didn't know enough to make a decision. Nevertheless, I was intrigued by what the woman said. Maybe this method would work for me? Maybe I didn't have to lose my breast after all? I now had another option.

Had I known more about alternative treatments, I might have seri-

Early Diagnosis and Treatment Can Save Your Life

ously considered it as a treatment option. Unfortunately, time was not on my side. It was too late to do any research. So, by the time I'd gotten home, I was back on track. I had made my decision.

My co-workers were very supportive of me, especially Dena. Another one belonged to a prayer group on campus. She told me they prayed for me at every prayer meeting. I was so touched by her love and support. Another recommended all kinds of books to read that might help me better understand healing from a spiritual standpoint. I'd read several articles on the importance of being in good physical and emotional shape before surgery. I was determined to do all I could do to maximize my chances of surviving the disease. First, I had to get past the surgery.

I prayed more in those last two days prior to surgery than I had ever prayed my entire life. I knew I really needed God to take this battle. I could not do it; I wasn't strong enough. Finally, the night before the surgery, I relinquished all ownership and power this disease had over me. It was only then a sense of peace and calm replaced the spiritual chaos.

Nathan arrived at my house around 6:15 a.m. Saturday morning. I had already showered and was just enjoying the stillness of the morning. I asked him to lie down with me for a few minutes. He held me really close. It was so quiet, quiet enough to hear the sound of our heartbeats. Neither one of us said a word. After what seemed like a long time, I got dressed. I went to Michelle's room and said goodbye to her.

My surgery was scheduled for 8:00 a.m. Nathan accompanied me to registration. We were led to another floor where I was escorted to a room so that I could change. I was glad he was upbeat. Maybe he was putting up a good front for me. I was hoping that he had said a prayer for me too. He waited in the room with me until the nurse came to get me. It was time.

I was put in a wheelchair and wheeled down to another room. I was immediately placed on a bed and prepped for surgery. I said one more prayer:

"God please guide the surgeons' hands; let the cancer only be in my left breast. Please bless and keep me as I have this surgery. Thank You for all that you've done, that You're doing, and that You are going to do in my life. Let your will be done. In your precious Son Jesus' name, Amen."

One nurse started the IV while another checked all the instruments that were placed on the table just to my left. I could tell that the sedative was beginning to work because I started getting very sleepy. The last thing I remember was seeing Dr. George.

The surgery lasted nearly six hours and I had been in the recovery room about two hours. One of the nurses came to my bedside and said I had come through the surgery like a champ. I was still somewhat drowsy from the medication, but I did notice several tubes and a very large bandage across the left side of my chest. I thought it might feel a little lighter since they had removed a 40D-sized breast. The nurse who was caring for me was very patient and professional, not anything like the horror stories I'd heard regarding patient care at Kaiser Hospital. She made sure I was comfortable and had enough pain medication. Moments later, Dr. George entered the recovery room.

"The surgery went fine, Nicole," she said as she gave me a reassuring pat on my right shoulder. Some of your family members are downstairs in the waiting area. I've already talked to them. They will be allowed to come to see you once you're taken to your room."

Even in my sedated state, Dr. George made me feel better. I managed a smile of approval. A tear rolled down the side of my face. I closed my eyes and thanked God for getting me through the surgery.

I was taken to my room. My sister, Barbara, and her friend Charlotte were there. Several bouquets of flowers had been delivered. The nurse skillfully maneuvered the wheelchair that carried me around the chairs and parked it next to the bed.

"How you feeling?" Barbara asked.

"I don't know. It's too early to tell. The only thing I know right now is that my titty's gone," I said, still light-headed.

"Hi, Nikki," Charlotte said very softly.

I didn't feel much like conversation and I'm sure they knew it, so they both agreed to come back later that evening. While one nurse assisted me into the bed, another wheeled in what resembled a small portable computer box. She began to enter some numbers in the machine and when she finished the nurse rolled the apparatus over to my bed and handed me a small hand-held attachment.

"Ms. Bryant, this machine has been programmed so you can get

Early Diagnosis and Treatment Can Save Your Life

your pain medication as you need it. Just press the button whenever you think you feel pain. The medication will be released automatically, in preset dosages," the nurse instructed me.

"What medication?" I asked drowsily.

"It's morphine," she answered.

I slept several more hours and awoke to the aroma of green pepper shrimp fried rice. Michelle and JuJu had come by to visit and brought my favorite Chinese food dish. I hadn't eaten anything since late Friday night and was starving. I didn't realize the effect eating so quickly after surgery would have on me. I had no sooner finished my meal when I threw up everything. I was sicker than ever. I felt so bad for them because they were trying to help, but instead made things worse. Once I got cleaned up, they left. By now it was almost 8:00 in the evening and I was still exhausted from the lengthy procedure.

By Sunday morning, the effects of the anesthesia had completely worn off, and the realization of my breastlessness hit me. While I was glad to know the cancerous breast had been removed, I had already begun to feel the weight of my loss. Dr. George arrived early that morning. She examined the incision, removed the large mounds of cloth and bandages, and replaced it with a much smaller piece of gauze and bandages. She inspected the drainage tubes that ran from the surgery site to a small pouch, being careful not to dislodge them.

"The tubes and drainage will probably be removed tomorrow, and if all goes well, you'll probably be able to go home on Tuesday morning."

"That would be great!"

Even though I'd been hospitalized for only a few days, I was glad my stay would be short. One of my biggest concerns was that there would be some complications or the cancer had spread. The result would have meant a longer hospital stay.

The small pouch was somewhat of a nuisance and the tubes got in the way. Because the surgery was on my left side and the IV was on my right side, just lying in bed was a challenge. The only position that gave me a little comfort was on my back. I didn't realize the magnitude of the surgery. I thought that just my left side would be affected. Instead, I couldn't use either arm with any effectiveness. Getting in and out of bed to use the bathroom

Early Diagnosis and Treatment Can Save Your Life

was an even greater hurdle. I absolutely refused to use that awful bedpan. I was helpless and self-pity began to creep in. I cried a lot between visitors.

My family and friends had been great. A few of them visited but were mindful that I was recovering from major surgery and needed to rest. They made sure I had plenty to eat, visited in shifts, assisted the nurses with me, and called regularly. It would have been easy to milk this situation, but of course I didn't. And, as promised, Nathan visited several times.

Dr. George came by early Monday morning. She performed a thorough examination, replaced the old bandages with new ones, and removed the drainage tubes. This gave me a little bit more mobility on my left side.

"Everything looks good, Nicole. You can go home tomorrow."

I was elated; my prayers had been answered.

Nathan arrived at the hospital shortly after Dr. George left. I was feeling much better and eager to tell him that I would be going home. He brought flowers and a card, and always had a big smile on his face. He sat with me until he had to go to work. Most of my family and a few co-workers came by also. By midday, my room was bursting with flowers, cards, and other gifts. The nursing staff at the hospital had very little to do for me because my friends and family helped out a great deal. I was accustomed to doing everything for myself or helping other people so it felt strange having everyone doting on me.

I told everyone who visited that I was going to be released the next day. Nathan came by two more times that day. On his last visit, he helped me put my clothes and personal items into my suitcase. I was ready to go home. I should have known that things were going too well to be true. By the time Nathan left the hospital that night, I was really fatigued. I just assumed it was my body's reaction to having major surgery and having a lot of visitors. I crawled into bed and quickly drifted to sleep.

I awoke around 3:00 a.m. with my gown completely soaked. The sheets were so saturated I thought I had wet the bed. Just as I tried to get out of the bed, the night nurse entered my room. She could see something was wrong and immediately called for assistance. As my mother would say, I was as weak as a three-day-old kitten. I could barely lift my body. The two nurses put me in the chair next to my bed. While one of the nurses changed the linen, the other took my temperature. It was 102.5. Even though sweat

Early Diagnosis and Treatment Can Save Your Life

dripped off me as if I had just exited from the depths of hell, my body was ice-cold. The nurse called Dr. George to inform her of my condition. I don't know what exactly Dr. George told her to do, but the nurse exited the room, while the other assisted me in changing my nightgown. The other nurse returned a short time later with some medication.

"Ms. Bryant, this should help bring the fever down."

I took the pills and was led back to my dry bed.

The nurses checked my temperature periodically throughout the night. By the time Dr. George made her rounds Tuesday morning, my temperature slightly dropped. She inspected the site where the drainage tubes had been removed. It didn't appear to have an infection. An order was placed to have my blood drawn for testing. Because I still had a slight temperature, the doctor did not release me.

She also informed me she would not be in for a few days and that another doctor would be making her rounds. I didn't like that another doctor would be taking over my care, even if only for a few days. I had become so accustomed and comfortable with Dr. George. But, what could I do?

My temperature stayed pretty stable all that day and most of the night, but by early Wednesday morning I awoke to a wet bed, chills, and sweats. When the nurse took my temperature, it was 102.9. All the bedding was changed and I was given clean sleepwear and medication to control the fever.

When the two new doctors came to examine me, my temperature still hovered in the mid 101's.

"I see you've had a rough couple of nights," the older doctor commented as he picked up my chart.

The other doctor, a young African American male who appeared to be not much older than my son, came over to inspect the surgery site. He smiled as he carefully removed the old bandages.

"You're going to do a doctor proud; the incision looks really good."

"Well, I'm glad that you like the scar and hopefully when you come by tomorrow, I will feel as good as the scar looks," I replied.

I'm sure it was just his good bedside manner, but I could have sworn he was flirting with me (no doubt I was hallucinating from the fever). I

Early Diagnosis and Treatment Can Save Your Life

know that flirting was the furthest thing from this doctor's mind, but it sure made me feel better even pretending he was. Besides, I'd had a breast removed, not my eyes. He was so cute.

I managed to put on a smile, trying to be as pleasant as I could under the circumstances. The handsome young doctor replaced the bandages then picked up my chart and made a few notations. The doctors moved to the foot of the bed and quietly discussed my chart. The older one told me that Dr. George would be back the next day to see me. I was hoping one of them would say something about the persistent fevers. Without giving me an explanation, they moved on to their next patient.

Not only was I getting bored with being in the hospital, but I was also growing more nervous about my health. I was becoming increasingly restless because not only did I not know what was wrong with me, but also the doctors didn't appear to know. It was frustrating that I had come through the actual surgery without any problems; yet, the fever would keep me in the hospital. It was my fifth day, and I was ready to go home. I wanted to sleep in my own queen-sized bed, in my own house, between my own covers. I missed my grandchildren terribly.

Nathan came by almost every day I was in the hospital, three times a day, and this was no exception…this was his third trip. He was there so much that one of the nurses made a sign to put on the door. It read, "Mister's in the House, Do Not Disturb." On one occasion, she even suggested that he could spend the night. I think she was impressed with how attentive he was.

I was in somewhat of a funk when Nathan came by that evening. I had grown increasingly weary about my condition. I needed a hug.

"Come and lay with me," I asked him.

"Are you sure?"

"Yeah, I'm very sure."

He took his shoes off and snuggled up very close to me. We barely fit on the small bed. I asked him to get under the covers. My body pressed up against his and I could feel him becoming aroused.

"I'm not hurting you, am I?"

"No, I'm fine. Go close the door," I whispered.

He hesitated at first, but then agreed. He closed the door, leaving

Early Diagnosis and Treatment Can Save Your Life

just enough opening to see out. He got back into the bed. It felt good having him next to me. He always smelled so good. Nathan was an excellent kisser. What started out very innocent turned into something more than we both had planned. With bandages, stitches, limited mobility, morphine tank, IV in one arm, and that small bed, we made love. Nathan was especially gentle, being careful not to hurt me. Fortunately for us, no one came into the room. As far as I know, they may have even guessed what we were doing and allowing us time to be alone. Nathan stayed with me for quite a while. He must have quietly slipped away while I was asleep, because I don't even remember him leaving.

I was awakened in the middle of night by the coolness of the bed. My fever was up higher than it had previously been, to 103.7. I was now getting scared, and for the first time I could see from the looks on the nurses' faces they were worried also.

Dr. George made her usual early morning rounds to my room. Concern swept her face. She examined the area around the drainage area and the surgery site. Nothing was apparent to justify the fevers. She walked to the end of the bed, picked up my chart and made some notations on it. She put it down and came back to the head of the bed.

"Nicole, I am concerned about the fevers. There doesn't appear to be an infection and all the blood work taken so far has come back negative. I don't know what's causing the elevated temperatures. Usually, when a person has a fever, the white cell count goes up as a way to combat the infection. But in your case, the cells aren't going up, nor are they going down. It's as if your body doesn't know it has a fever. I'm going to have someone from the Infectious Disease Control Unit talk to you."

The words "Infectious Disease Control" struck a nerve. The only thing that immediately came to my mind was HIV and AIDS.

"Have you ever been tested for HIV or AIDS?" she asked.

"No," I replied solemnly.

"I'm going to order you to be tested; we have to rule everything out. Someone will come up later today."

Dr. George exited my room. I was in a trance-like state, overcome with a fear like I'd never felt. It never occurred to me that something else more serious could be wrong. AIDS was the furthest thing from my

Early Diagnosis and Treatment Can Save Your Life

mind. I kept thinking to myself, "God would not do this to me—breast cancer and AIDS. He would not be this cruel."

While the fear was overwhelming, it didn't take long before fear turned into anger, and anger quickly disintegrated into feelings of helplessness and hopelessness. I lay there thinking about my sexual partners. I'd been careful, particularly in the past several years. The mere thought of having AIDS on top of breast cancer was too much for me to bear.

Once the initial shock of possibly having another deadly disease wore off, I became angry, angry to the point of thinking of killing anyone who I thought may have infected me. I started with George because I'd been with him the longest. As far as I knew, he had no serious illnesses. I swore if he'd given me anything, I was going to kill him when I got out of the hospital.

I spent most of the day worrying about my new predicament. Had I carelessly put my health, and maybe my life, in danger? Could it be Nathan? As far as I knew he was okay, but then again, how did I really know if he was safe? We'd been careful up until that night by the side of the road. How could I have been so careless? I know it only takes one time. Even if Nathan was the culprit, it would have been too soon for the disease to show up. I had to consider past relationships, those ten to fifteen years ago. This was self-imposed torture. Between the fevers, worrying about having AIDS, crying, and planning my revenge, my day was pretty miserable. I know this was not the time to be thinking evil, but nothing mattered except that if I was going to die, I was going to take someone with me.

The doctor from Infectious Disease came by later that afternoon. She looked at my chart and told me that someone would arrive to take some blood. She told me that Dr. George had requested a rush on the test and the results would be back in about two days. While the doctor was there, a nurse brought in some papers for me to sign so they could administer the HIV/AIDS test.

My sister Dorothy called and I told her what was going on. She tried to reassure me I didn't have AIDS and I shouldn't worry about it. If I had had HIV/AIDS, she surmised, they would have discovered it

Early Diagnosis and Treatment Can Save Your Life

when they took all my blood work prior to the surgery. While her reassurance was comforting, this little voice of self-doubt kept wondering "what if?" I had made it through one battle, the breast cancer; now I had to prepare myself for the annihilation—AIDS.

The next morning was uneventful. Nathan made his usual daily visit, but his stay was brief. I asked him not to come back later because I was scheduled to have several more tests. He reluctantly agreed.

Later that night, the fever was just as high as the night before. With the possibility of AIDS looming over my head, I was an emotional wreck. The fear was paramount. I was convinced I was going to die. I never thought I would ever welcome breast cancer, but compared to having AIDS, I secretly did.

The nurse who had come to change my linens could tell I was upset.

"Are you okay, Ms. Bryant?"

"Not really. The doctors can't seem to find out why I keep having a fever, so they are testing me for HIV and AIDS."

"Ms. Bryant, you don't have HIV or AIDS because if you did, you would be showing some signs."

"Really?" I responded, unconvinced.

"Yeah," she continued. "When a woman has HIV or AIDS there are some obvious signs. It's hard for her not to know something's wrong."

"Like what?" I asked.

"One of the signs is a thick yellowish discharge that smells horrible. Trust me, Ms. Bryant, if you had HIV or AIDS you would know it by now. You're gonna be all right."

"I hope so."

She finished with the covers and helped me back into the bed. I felt a little bit relieved. When I prayed that night, I not only asked God to spare me from another disease, but I also asked Him to forgive me for my sins and to forgive me for every bad thought I'd had.

The next two days were gut-wrenching. Waiting for the results was bad enough, but anticipating what the test results would reveal was agonizing. I wasn't really up to having visitors; however, I put on a brave face as if all was okay. The usual parade of family and friends came by, including Nathan. I could have received an Academy Award for my

Early Diagnosis and Treatment Can Save Your Life

bedside performance. No one even suspected I was going through another crisis.

The results were back. I knew when Dr. George entered the room it was good news. I know doctors aren't supposed to show much emotion, but Dr. George was different from any physician I'd ever had, which was one of the reasons I liked her so much.

"The tests were negative, Nicole."

"Thank you, God. Thank you, thank you, thank you," I cried out.

"We still don't know what's causing the fevers," Dr. George lamented. "I guess your body just doesn't like the trauma of the surgery because we can't find anything. All the tests that we've done so far have come back negative. We're going to watch you very closely for a day or so to see if the fever breaks. If it doesn't, we'll run more tests."

I didn't care anymore that they couldn't figure out what was causing the fevers. The only thing that mattered was I didn't have HIV or AIDS. I could even deal with a few more uncomfortable nights of discomfort. I had just received two blessings from God and I wasn't about to let anything take away my joy.

Unfortunately, the fevers persisted; however, the temperatures weren't as elevated as they had been—now running in the low 100's.

Finally, the fevers seemed to have broken. Despite still being slightly raised, Dr. George said I could go home.

I had become bored to death of TV, reading, the hospital bed, and watching the soaps, but more than anything, I had grown very weary of the smell of medicine and of sickness. I was so ready to get back to my home, my family, my job, my life. I arrived at Kaiser Hospital on Saturday, October 29, expecting to go home in a few days; instead, I was released November 11, some fourteen days later.

In a strange sort of way, the hospital became my refuge. While there, I did not have to feel, think, or wonder what I was going to do next and how I was going to do it. These next few days were going to be critical. Would I be able to handle the 'new' me and all the stuff that awaited outside of these hospital walls?

Dr. George came by to make one final check before officially discharging me.

Early Diagnosis and Treatment Can Save Your Life

"I can't wait to get home so I can start walking the lake again," I said as Dr. George completed her final exam.

"I don't want you doing any activity until after your follow-up appointment with me. The only place I want you to walk, young lady, is from your bedroom to the bathroom and kitchen, that's it. Nothing strenuous, no long walks. Absolutely no lifting or pulling with your left arm. I want you to take it easy over the next couple of weeks," Dr. George insisted.

Armed with Dr. George's pager numbers, emergency numbers, patient help line number, and a thermometer, I was discharged. Post-surgery care instructions were as follows: Driving, no. Bathing, yes. Lifting, no. Stairs, yes. Sexual relations, yes. She could have put "no" by the sex as well. In light of my AIDS scare, it was the furthest thing from my mind. Because my stay in the hospital had been longer than anticipated, the drains, tubing, and staples had all been removed, so I didn't have all that to worry about. My discharge order included the date of my first post-surgery appointment with Dr. George and my appointment to see the oncologist. It was obvious I was going to be busy with doctor visits for the next several weeks. By the time all the paperwork was completed for my release, it was around 10:30 a.m. Michelle picked me up from the hospital and I was on my way home.

The ride was short, but positively invigorating. For the first time in weeks, I breathed fresh air. Everything seemed new, but refreshingly familiar. Even the brown palm trees looked good.

Michelle and I had a lot of catching up to do. I was looking forward to seeing Briannah and Jerica. They were so young and didn't quite understand all of what was happening to their NaNa, but the one thing they did know is that their NaNa had to get one of her tittys cut off. They had given me so much joy and laughter in the short time they had been on this earth. It's amazing how much of my recovery and will to live was attributed to their little lives.

Thanksgiving was just a few weeks away, so being home meant a great deal to me. I didn't know what was in store, but I asked God to watch over me, give me understanding, and help me get through it. I knew He had brought me through a lot and didn't bring me that far to

Early Diagnosis and Treatment Can Save Your Life

leave me. I felt ready for any challenge that would come my way. I had so much for which to be thankful.

Early Diagnosis and Treatment Can Save Your Life

For I will restore your health onto thee, and I will heal thee of thy wounds, saith the Lord.

Jeremiah 30:17

5

One Titty Gone

Being in the hospital did have its advantages (like being waited on hand and foot and having someone available for my every beck and call), but I was sure glad to be home. For the first night in fourteen days I was sleeping in my bed, waking up to the sound of my favorite radio station, while in familiar surroundings with their usual aromas. It was absolutely divine. No more daily doctor visits, no more needles, no more of those awful hospital gowns, no more blood tests. My first day back was pretty much the same as it had been in the hospital. Most of my family came by and my phone rang constantly. And yes, Nathan was there. He continued to be very supportive.

Several days after arriving home, I received a call from an American Cancer Society (ACS) representative. The Breast Care Coordinator at Kaiser Hospital had given my name to them. She greatly detailed ACS's programs and wanted to assign me a Reach To Recovery Volunteer who was a breast cancer survivor. I asked if the volunteer could be an African American woman. I needed to know and interact with another African American woman who had gone through what I was about to experience.

I decided to accept her offer for the volunteer to come see me. The Reach to Recovery volunteer called me the next morning and my appointment was scheduled for that same day. I realized how much I needed to talk to someone who could understand some of my fears and issues, and to just be able to share some of what I was going through with someone who had already been through it.

Prior to that phone conversation, I had only heard the term "breast cancer survivor" on one other occasion when I talked to Gillie. I didn't know what I considered myself. I had just survived the surgery and the hospital stay. It was too soon to determine if I'd actually survived the cancer. But knowing there were other African American women who had survived this disease was encouraging to say the least. It gave me

Early Diagnosis and Treatment Can Save Your Life

hope, and hope was something I desperately needed.

In the few days I was home, I had already begun to experience an array of emotions. I wasn't sure if I could survive my own feelings of inadequacy and my anxiety about my mortality. I felt like a statistic, a casualty of this insidious war called breast cancer.

My door bell rang promptly at 12:30 that afternoon. I was surprised to see a young woman, much younger than myself, at the door. She greeted me with a big hug, which let me know I could feel comfortable with her. Jackie was a very friendly, articulate African American woman, who, at the time that I met her, was a five-year breast cancer survivor. She was in her late twenties when she was diagnosed with breast cancer. Like me, Jackie had a mastectomy.

What struck me most about Jackie was her willingness to share her most intimate thoughts about the disease. She had also gone through reconstruction surgery. I didn't know reconstruction surgery was an option for me. Maybe in the madness I was told about it, but I never gave it serious consideration before meeting Jackie.

"Could I see your reconstructed breast?" I asked.

"Sure," she said as she began to unbutton her blouse.

She pulled her blouse back and unfastened her bra. There it was, her reconstructed breast, complete with areola, nipple, and just enough contour to look natural. Her new mound of flesh fascinated me. I never thought I would get this excited over another woman's breast, but I was ecstatic.

"Wow, it looks so real, can I feel it?"

"Yeah, you can touch it," she said.

I gently touched her breast.

"It even feels real. I don't care what it takes, I want one just like it," I joked.

She laughed, and for the first time in weeks, I had a good laugh too. We talked for hours.

Hearing about other women with this disease was one thing; meeting someone younger than me who actually lived to tell her story was absolutely incredible. Meeting her made me aware of things I hadn't even considered. She made me aware breast cancer was not some rare

Early Diagnosis and Treatment Can Save Your Life

disease among African American women. Jackie's visit also made me realize I still had a long way to go in terms of my overall well-being, both physically and emotionally. There was so much more I had to learn about my disease, and about myself. I was glad to have met this young, beautiful woman, who not only survived, but also appeared to be coping very well. I wanted to be where she was.

When she left, I looked through the goody bag she'd brought me. There was plenty of literature to read. One of the items in the bag was a pouch filled with cotton that I could use to stuff inside my bra until I got fitted for my prosthesis. The opening in the pouch was for inserting more cotton if needed. In my case, lots more cotton would be needed to match my right breast.

It had been weeks since I'd worn a bra and I was anxious to see what I looked like. I put on one of my bras and stuffed the pouch inside. It left a lot to be desired; however, it did give the appearance that there was at least something on the left side of my chest. The thought of wearing that pouch convinced me that I needed reconstruction.

During my first follow-up appointment, Dr. George told me I could take as long as I needed to stay off work to recuperate. I decided that I was ready to return to my job. My family, friends, and Dr. George thought I was crazy for rushing back so quickly, but I honestly felt that I could handle it. I had pretty much made up my mind I wasn't going to allow this disease to dictate my life, but I wasn't quite sure how I was going to go about doing it. I did know that I didn't want to stay at home another day. I needed to get back to the life I had before breast cancer interrupted it.

After being home just one week from the hospital, I went back to work. It felt good getting back to my usual routine. It allowed me to think about other things besides breast cancer. However, I quickly discovered that dealing with the physical pain of breast cancer wasn't nearly as bad as all the emotional pain.

My co-workers seemed to be both relieved and concerned at my returning so quickly after being released from the hospital. I'm sure Dena and the other females were comfortable with me, but I could sense my male co-worker seemed somewhat uneasy. I wanted everyone to

Early Diagnosis and Treatment Can Save Your Life

feel at ease and I certainly didn't want them to treat me any differently or make a fuss over me.

The first hour or so was kind of awkward. I needed to break the ice. "Okay, listen up everybody."

They all stopped what they were doing.

"I don't want to be treated any differently than I was before the surgery. I'm okay. I had a breast removed. Not my hands, my legs, my eyes, and not my brain. I'm still the same Nicole, just minus one insignificant body part." (My sense of humor was still intact).

I thanked them for their prayers and support and then reassured them that it was okay for me to be back. It lightened the atmosphere and we were all quickly back to the work and the business at hand.

Since I couldn't start walking right away, I was riding the bus to and from work. Nathan was driving another route so he arrived at my house around 6:30 p.m. every day. It was like old times, except that I was now dealing with my feelings of inadequacy and insecurities. I never once considered what impact my breast removal would have on my sexuality or how it would affect my overall well-being. Nor had I considered how he would feel. Other than my telling him that I had breast cancer, we hadn't discussed it anymore. I wasn't even comfortable talking about the disease, let alone discussing it with him. Aside from the unplanned sexual encounter in the hospital, Nathan and I hadn't been intimate. I was okay with that and glad he hadn't tried to initiate anything again. I realized I wasn't ready yet.

Several more weeks passed. This particular day, Nathan picked me up from work. No one was home when we arrived and it was kind of nice to have the house to ourselves. So, we thought that it was a perfect time to seize the moment. I slipped into the cute, little, short paisley print robe that my girlfriend, Heather, bought me when I was in the hospital. We sat on my bed talking for a long time, mostly about football. I talked very briefly about my visit with Jackie and that I was considering breast reconstruction.

Before long, kissing, rubbing, and patting ensued. Soon I was on my back with him lying gently on top of me. He was so concerned that he would hurt me that we laid on our sides. We were almost there. Then

Early Diagnosis and Treatment Can Save Your Life

I heard the front door open. We had just enough time to straighten our clothes and compose ourselves. Nathan and I sat on the side of the bed—trying to pretend we were doing something other than what we were about to do—as if we were sixteen-year-olds who had just gotten caught by their parents.

"Hey Mom," Michelle yelled out, as she entered the door.

She then greeted Nathan.

"Mom, what is that thing sticking out of your clothes?" she asked, as she came closer to inspect it.

"What's what?" I asked.

She pointed to the cotton pouch. Unbeknownst to me, it had wormed its way out of my bra and was resting conspicuously under my chin. In my haste to collect myself, I didn't see it come out. It was embarrassing enough for my daughter to see; I would have been crushed if Nathan had seen it. Then again, maybe he did and pretended he didn't.

"How in the world did that get there?" I asked, as I quickly shoved it back in my bra.

Michelle and I burst into laughter. Even though it was an uncomfortable situation, I could appreciate the humor in it. Nathan and I quickly realized this was not the right time for us to indulge in anything other than good conversation.

We didn't even try to make love again. Besides, I wasn't feeling particularly desirable. More than anything, I wasn't ready for him to see my body. I was very careful not to let Nathan see me undress or without my gown or robe and I always wore a t-shirt under my clothing. I felt naked without it—it became my armor.

I wasn't sure if my feelings were typical. I figured I would work through this, and when the time was right, nature would take its course. I was eager to regain my self confidence and find my way back to being the passionate, uninhibited woman I once was.

My physical scars were healing and becoming less visible, but my emotional scars were still raw. Once again, my breasts were dictating my perception femininity and sexuality, but for far different reasons than in the past. Consequently, having sex took a back seat; cuddling,

Early Diagnosis and Treatment Can Save Your Life

holding, and touching, coupled with long passionate kisses, became the norm.

Since leaving the hospital, I had not looked at my body in the mirror. I wasn't prepared to see my body without my breast so I avoided them. When I showered, I would place my towel on the curtain rod so that I could immediately wrap myself in it. The mirror in the bathroom extended over the entire wall, so I made sure I was completed covered when I emerged. I would quickly retreat to my bedroom, dry myself off, put lotion on my body, and put on my underwear without looking into a mirror. I knew this made absolutely no sense.

Breast cancer ultimately forces you to face acceptance—it was time. I finally found the courage to stand in front of the mirror to really look, to examine this new body.

I exited to shower and kept the towel around me until I made my way to my bedroom. I made sure that the bedroom door was locked because I didn't want Briannah or Michelle coming into my room. I stood in front of the mirror and slowly opened the towel.

The first thing I noticed was how large my right breast appeared. It was huge and seemed to hang down to my knees (of course it didn't, but that was my perception at that moment). My eyes moved to my now-barren left side. The incision stretched from the inside of my chest to under my arm, just past my shoulder blade. The skin where my breast had been was now tight and jagged. Several indentations remained from where the drainage tubes had been removed. Dark scars replaced my once smooth brown skin. I stood there for a few moments staring at my mutilated chest.

My thoughts sliced the silence.

"I'll be damned, my titty is gone. It's really gone."

Tears obscured my reflection in the mirror. It was too late to change my mind about having the mastectomy. I wished I had thought about it more. I wished that I could go back to a time when life wasn't so cruel.

I turned sideways to the left and then to the right side, thinking how unreal this all seemed. Maybe I should have had both of them removed; at least both sides of my chest would have matched. There was nothing beautiful about my chest. This new body looked ugly, strange,

Early Diagnosis and Treatment Can Save Your Life

deformed. I desperately tried to remember images of my former self; a lost memory I knew I couldn't recapture. What I would have given to have that inverted nipple again.

Early Diagnosis and Treatment Can Save Your Life

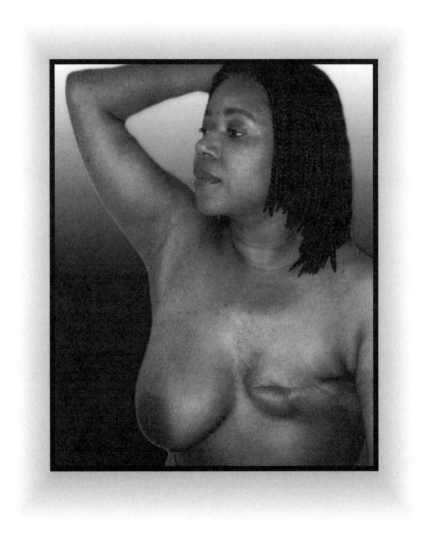

Early Diagnosis and Treatment Can Save Your Life

> *Be strong and of good courage, fear not, nor be afraid of them: for the Lord thy God, He it is that doth go with thee; He will not fail thee, nor forsake thee.*
>
> **Deuteronomy 31:6**

Early Diagnosis and Treatment Can Save Your Life

6

The Phantom Breast Blues

While I reached a milestone that day, I didn't know if I could handle this new chest, but I reluctantly accepted my disfigured body. This repackaged self was going to bring some challenges. I was reminded of all those years I'd prayed that my left breast could be different. Be careful what you pray for and what you put out there in the universe; you may get what you ask for. You may not necessarily get it how you want it, but you'll get it. In my case, that's exactly what happened. I spent years worrying about my left breast, even thought about surgery to correct it. Well, surgery did correct my breast; it just wasn't the correction I anticipated. It's ironic it took breast cancer to make my breast "better." Given my past feelings about my body when it WAS free of disease, I knew that I would have even bigger issues with this "new" one.

At least the holiday season would give me a respite from my anxieties. Holidays were big events for us. The entire family gathered at Dorothy's house for Thanksgiving. We would pick the name of the person to exchange a Christmas gift. Christmas was usually spent at Barbara's house and New Year's at mine, a tradition in our family for more than twenty years.

Thanksgiving came, and, as expected, everyone had a good time. It was an especially emotional time for me because I had lived to celebrate it. The smell of pies and different aromas from all the foods were more distinct. The food tasted better, the kids seemed to enjoy themselves more, and having all my friends and family around, can be described as one thing – precious. Gratitude took on a whole new meaning. The saying, 'not being promised tomorrow' really hit home for me. I didn't know if I'd be around to celebrate another one.

At the Thanksgiving gathering, I announced to the family that I wanted to have Christmas at my house. I didn't give any reason for doing it and no one asked me why, but deep down inside, I was afraid this could possibly be the last Christmas I would spend with them. I wanted it to be extra special.

Early Diagnosis and Treatment Can Save Your Life

My next follow-up visit with Dr. George went very well. The physical scars were on the mend. Emotionally, I was still very fragile. I still kept a lot of what I was feeling inside. I probably should have talked to her, or somebody, about my feelings, but didn't. I received a clean bill of health so it was all that really mattered to me.

My appointment to see the oncologist was next. I didn't do a lot of thinking about the possibility of receiving chemotherapy. What little I had read wasn't good, and what I'd heard was even worse. Just the thought of it was downright scary. Poison kills, and I had read enough to know that chemo was poison. When I first learned I had breast cancer, Dr. George mentioned chemotherapy as a possible preventive measure. I accepted that if I died of the disease, then so be it, but I wasn't going to put myself through rounds of chemo unless it was absolutely necessary. I knew chemo saved lives, but I was more concerned with the quality of my life. Since Dr. George didn't insist I receive it, in my mind, it wasn't a definite for me. I was leaning more towards not having the treatments.

When I arrived at the oncologist's office I was feeling strong and prepared to make a decision about my treatment option. I was escorted back to a large room that looked as if it served as a meeting room as well as a doctor's office. The doctor entered.

"Oh, Ms. Bryant, you're here," he said, as if my visit surprised him.

I was somewhat troubled by his greeting. It almost seemed as if he didn't expect me. Initially, I thought I might be overly sensitive; that this might have been his way of greeting all his patients.

Two young blond ladies accompanied him. By their attire, they appeared to be doctors as well. He introduced them to me, saying they were visiting interns from overseas. There was a small table in his office and several chairs were in front of his desk. The two young ladies sat at the table as if to observe the doctor and me. I assumed the very thick medical file on his desk was mine.

"Have a seat, Ms. Bryant, and give me a moment," the oncologist said, as he pointed to one of the chairs in front of the desk.

The doctor opened my file, which was approximately four inches thick, turned the pages, and ran his fingers through the information as if he were speed reading.

Early Diagnosis and Treatment Can Save Your Life

"Uh uh, okay, uh uh," he mumbled, as he turned the pages.

In less than twenty seconds he closed my file and was ready to give his recommendation.

The doctor's lack of preparation disturbed me. I was there to make what probably was the most important decision of my life and he appeared to not be as serious about it as I thought he should be. While it didn't seem to be a big deal to him, this visit was paramount for me.

"Now," he said casually.

I watched in disbelief as he closed my file.

It was one thing the doctor didn't even have the decency to review my file prior to my arrival, but when he hastily read over it as if he were skimming through the morning newspaper, I was outraged and insulted. I had been to enough doctors to know this was not how a patient's medical file should be reviewed, or should a diagnosis be made based on a quick glance of the information.

He proceeded to give me a lot of statistical information about African American women and breast cancer, never once really relating to me on an individual basis. I told him that I wasn't a statistic, didn't appreciate being treated like one, and that I wanted an opinion based on my personal history and not on a bunch of numbers.

What was even more unsettling than his giving me his opinion about the chemotherapy treatment was that he actually thought I would take his advice. When I told him I wasn't going to make the decision right away, he appeared annoyed with me. He insisted he needed to have my decision within the next few days so he could make arrangements to start the treatments. I told him I wasn't prepared to make such a major decision at that time and that I needed to discuss it with my family and especially my sister, who was a nurse. He appeared to become even more annoyed.

Prior to visiting the oncologist, I was leaning towards not having the treatments. When I left that doctor's office, I was one hundred percent certain I wasn't going to have it. I took it as God's way of letting me know I would be okay without the chemotherapy. I left the doctor's office feeling empowered and in control of my destiny. I was okay with my decision. Just as I'd done with all my other decisions, I prayed and

Early Diagnosis and Treatment Can Save Your Life

asked God for guidance, and that I would accept His will. There is no better feeling than making a decision based on your trust and faith in Him.

In between my job and doctor visits, I managed to prepare for Christmas. I wanted it to be memorable just in case it would be my last one with my family. The college's two-week break gave me some much needed time.

I rented tables, chairs, and food warmers. The house was decorated throughout in green and red ornaments. The tree was large and overflowed with gifts. I bought something for everyone in the family, nearly thirty in all. Unlike our Thanksgiving feast where my family relieved me of cooking duties, I was strong enough to prepare some of the food. Of course, my sisters were quick to remind me I shouldn't be doing too much, so I was careful to pace myself.

My mother was making her usual Christmas visit. This would be the first time I'd seen her since my diagnosis. It was important for me that she got to see me healthy and that I had, for the time being, beat this disease. Even though she never said it directly, I knew my mother prayed for me. I also knew she worried about losing another child. I wanted to do this for her more than I wanted to do this for me.

We had a great Christmas celebration. As it turned out, I survived that Christmas and I'm grateful to have celebrated many, many more. (It took me nearly five years to pay for the Christmas of 1994.) In addition to celebrating the birth of Christ, that Christmas held special meaning for me in that it symbolized my new beginning. I was more relaxed than I had been in months and so was my family. Christmas offered a brief but welcomed reprieve from my breast cancer odyssey.

During my next appointment with Dr. George, I informed her that I had decided not to have the chemotherapy. She didn't seem surprised, so I suspected she had an inkling. I told her that I'd thought about it long and hard, had prayed about it, and had given it to God. (I decided not to tell her about my experience with the oncologist.) She encouraged me to continue following her instructions for post-surgery care and said she respected my decision. She told me that I could start exercising my arm a little bit and gave me a sample of the exercises. I was glad I could start

Early Diagnosis and Treatment Can Save Your Life

taking short walks and could drive again, but she insisted that I not lift anything. The only exercise I'd been able to do in months was to get in and out of bed. I was looking forward to a new challenge.

We discussed other post-surgery treatment—possibly hormonal therapy— Tamoxifen. Since I was totally against receiving chemotherapy, I had to think about other options. I had an opportunity to do some reading on Tamoxifen as well as an alternative approach. Each had its benefits; however, the thing that scared me most about Tamoxifen was one of its potential side effects: an increased risk of endometrial (lining of the uterus) cancer. I decided to pursue the alternative approach.

Doctor appointments had become routine. As much as I enjoyed my visits with Dr. George, I was glad that I didn't have to see her for a while.

I plunged myself into learning as much as I could about vitamins and minerals, massage, organic foods, green tea, flax seed, you name it. If it had anything to do with staying healthy, I tried it. I stocked up on Vitamins E, B Complex, and C; Beta Carotene, Zinc, Selenium, Co-Enzyme Q10, and Aloe Vera juice. Whole Foods, The Food Mill, and the Lakeshore Natural Food Company became my havens.

My appointment with the Breast Care Coordinator was just another in the long list of post-surgery events. I'd seen Ms. Beckley several times immediately after my diagnosis so I was familiar with her. She gave me the name and telephone number of the place I could be fitted for my prosthesis. After returning home, I called the number. My appointment to see the owner of A Woman's Touch salon would not take place for several weeks later.

Nearly two months had passed since I returned to work and had settled into my old routine. I thought I was progressing well physically until, one Monday while sitting at my desk, I felt what I thought was some coffee that spilled on my blouse. As it turned out, I had started bleeding and my blouse was full of blood.

"I'm just going to go home and change and come right back," I told Dena.

"No, you aren't. I'm taking your ass to the hospital," Dena insisted.

We were off to Kaiser Hospital Emergency Room. As it turned out,

Early Diagnosis and Treatment Can Save Your Life

an area of the surgery site, which had not completely healed, caused the bleeding. It was a temporary, but minor setback. I frankly didn't realize the toll major surgery would have on my body and how long it would take for the incisions to heal. Not only was I told the surgery site would take a while to heal, but my body would take an even longer time to recover from the trauma of having a part removed. After this incident, I decided to slow down a bit. It made me realize that my complete recovery was going to take some time.

I was glad this day had finally arrived. I could stop stuffing my bras with socks, panties, washcloths, cotton, anything that made my breast appear natural. I didn't know what to expect, but I figured anything would probably be better than what I had.

I arrived at A Woman's Touch early. The owner, Carolyn, was a young white woman who was quite friendly and personable. Her shop brimmed with all types of scarves, wigs, and other items designed for breast cancer survivors. While not a survivor, she was very knowledgeable about breast cancer and breast prostheses. I had no idea what a breast prosthesis would look like or even if it would work for me. The only thing I knew was I was ready to try almost anything that could bring balance to my body.

We talked a little bit about her and the services she provided to breast cancer survivors. I told her of my challenge to make my breast look as natural as possible. I shared with her how while leaving Kaiser Hospital I noticed my reflection as I walked past the window. It was very noticeable how lopsided my left side appeared. I knew that if I noticed it, other people did also. I couldn't wait to get home and take all the stuffing out of my bra. Carolyn reassured me the prosthesis would bring balance to my chest and would appear more natural than what I was using.

She showed me a prototype. I put it in my bra and buttoned my blouse. Not only did it look natural, it was almost a perfect fit and felt like a breast. The prosthesis, made of this thick rubbery material, was smooth to the touch. It even had a small nipple on it. I laughed when I saw it. I would finally get the nipple I'd always wanted. Granted it wasn't real, but it wasn't inverted either.

Early Diagnosis and Treatment Can Save Your Life

"Wow, this is amazing," I said with great enthusiasm. "What will they think of next?"

I had to try on several sizes before we actually matched it exactly to that of my right breast.

It was now time to select the color. She showed me several shades of beige and pink; however, I didn't see anything that came remotely close to my skin color. Not honey, not cinnamon, not dark brown, not chestnut, not coffee, nothing. When I asked her if she had a darker color, she said she didn't. The only color even close to my skin tone was the tawny, and to make matters worse, she had to order it because she didn't keep tawny in stock.

I was glad to be getting the prosthesis, but I was disappointed the salon didn't carry, nor (according to Carolyn) did the manufacturers make any color darker than tawny. While I knew the prosthesis wasn't a real breast, it would have been nice to wear something that looked more like my own skin color. So I seized the opportunity to interject a little humor in the situation.

"How is it that they make penises in any shape, size and color, from the lightest shade of pink to the darkest shade of black, yet they can't come up with a breast form darker than tawny. I don't understand that."

Carolyn managed a smile. Certainly, I wasn't the first African American woman who had come to this salon for a prosthesis. Why weren't there any colors that matched my skin? Was I asking for too much? The problem wasn't all Carolyn's fault; manufacturers had to be held accountable also.

I made light of the situation, but I was more serious than Carolyn knew. She said she would see if she could get a darker color, but that it was unlikely. In addition to not having my color in stock, she didn't have one in my size. Because the prosthesis had to be ordered, she gave a pattern for a pouch to be sewn into my bra. I told her my Reach To Recovery volunteer had given me a temporary prosthesis of sorts to put in my bra. Carolyn suggested that in order to make it feel the same as the right breast, I try putting rice or beans in it. This would give more weight to it and hold it in place better. I knew she was trying to be helpful, but I wasn't about to put rice or beans in my bra. I imagined myself

Early Diagnosis and Treatment Can Save Your Life

walking down the street and the pouch bursting, with the rice and beans going everywhere. This suggestion was almost as ridiculous as my visit with the oncologist was unsettling.

It took nearly three weeks for the prosthesis to arrive, and as expected, it was tawny. I decided to give it a name. Naming it somehow made it seem a part of me. I thought back to when I was a little kid. Every penny I got went to buying Mary Jane candy. I liked the way the name Mary Jane sounded. So, Mary Jane was born.

During the months that followed, Mary Jane was used for a lot of different things. I used it as a paper weight. Once while kidding around with my sister, I unashamedly removed it from my bra and used it to beat her. My granddaughters used it to play catch. On one occasion they accidentally ripped it. They felt really bad they had torn their NaNa's titty. To make them feel better, I put a bandage on the area that had torn. I kept that bandage on Mary Jane so they could see it when I put it on.

Mainly, I used it for its intended purpose, a temporary breast form. I guess I didn't appreciate Mary Jane as much as I should have. I knew it was only a matter of time and I would have the real thing—almost. But until then, it served the purpose well. I could at least go without having to camouflage my body with large blouses and covering up with even bigger jackets.

Even with Mary Jane, I still felt uncomfortable undressing in front of other people. I'll never forget one particular incident when I disrobed at the gym and women peered at me. I often wondered if this was because they had never seen a mastectomy or if they felt sorry for me.

The only exception was my granddaughters. Their stares were that of a child's innocence and curiosity, unlike others that I had received. It was obvious they had talked about my situation among themselves.

"NaNa, when are you going to get your new titty?" they would ask in unison.

As the months passed, I felt a little bit more comfortable with my body. Nathan hadn't let up either. He still came by every single day, sometimes two and three times a day. I was flattered by all the attention. He often told me that he admired my strength. It didn't seem to me I had been particularly strong. Every time I turned around I was crying

Early Diagnosis and Treatment Can Save Your Life

about something. I didn't know anybody personally who had experienced breast cancer so I had no one to compare myself with or to judge my progress. I just took my recovery one day at a time and constantly prayed that God would keep me healthy and strong.

Nathan had been really patient with me and never once pressured me. As the months passed, I began thinking a lot about making love to him. I often wondered why he stuck by me. He was seven years younger than I, very handsome and probably could have had any young woman he wanted. Did he feel sorry for me or did he genuinely care? We never talked about it. For that matter, I didn't talk to anyone about anything, sex and intimacy being no exception. I probably should have discussed how I was feeling with him, but I didn't and he didn't pressure me into talking. I just hoped things would work out. My fear of rejection played a big part in my waiting so long to become intimate again. My human frailties allowed my insecurities to keep me from being as spontaneous as I had been in the past.

Inasmuch as I tried not to associate my breast (or the lack of) with having anything to do with my sexuality, it was hard to do when constantly barraged with images of "perfect" breasts. A young lady shared with me her sister succumbed to breast cancer because her boyfriend told her he didn't want a woman with one breast. I met another woman who told me she didn't allow her husband to touch her breasts since she had her lumpectomy. Breast cancer leaves you in a very fragile and sometimes desperate place. The constant tug of war you have with yourself about body image can sometimes be more overwhelming than the disease itself.

The complexities were agonizing. I was glad the cancer was out of my body, but there were many times when I mourned the loss of my breast. I wanted so badly to feel whole and in a safe place; but haunted by my feelings of inadequacy. I often wondered what Nathan thought about it. I would rationalize by telling myself that he shouldn't have a problem with it; I was the one missing a body part. I knew my beauty had nothing to do with whether I did or didn't have breasts; however, I needed to be reminded that I was beautiful in spite of them. I wish I had talked to him about how he felt and about my feelings.

Early Diagnosis and Treatment Can Save Your Life

The time finally came. I planned the evening down to the last detail. Very dim lights, good music, a little wine, and a nice little two-piece lingerie set. I decided on a two piece because at least I wouldn't have to expose my chest if I didn't want to. I was concerned about how my barren chest would feel against Nathan's. Would he be turned off by it? Would having one breast affect my spontaneity? I was hoping it wouldn't.

The one detail I couldn't quite seem to decide was what to do with Mary Jane. If I kept it on, that meant I would have to keep my bra on as well, making it uncomfortable for him to get to my good breast. If I didn't wear it, I would feel naked and uncomfortable. I decided not to wear it. For that night, it would remain in the drawer.

I was as nervous as I was my very first time. The room was lit just enough so that we could see each other's silhouettes. His kisses were so soft. We lay there on the bed just holding each other. Then he asked if he could touch my breast. He gently caressed it. I didn't realize until that moment just how much I'd missed having it touched. He then asked me if he could touch my left side. I hesitated for just a second, but allowed him to feel the mastectomy scar. He gently ran his hand across the incision, and then slowly pulled the gown back so that he could see my body.

"Can I kiss your scar?"

I wasn't prepared for this, but I reluctantly agreed. I didn't want to be touched there yet, but I desperately wanted him to know I was trying to make my way back to being myself. I had come a long way, but I knew I still wasn't to a point where I felt completely comfortable with my body.

Nathan made me feel beautiful, loved, and free. Free to enjoy this man who had given so much of his time to me over the past months. Free to give and receive pleasure without hesitation.

Early Diagnosis and Treatment Can Save Your Life

The Phantom Breast Blues

My breasts betrayed me from the very start.
Left me feeling insecure, unsatisfied, yearning down in my heart.
Wanting bigger breasts, better breasts; it was more than just a whim,
Convinced Mother Nature could have done a better job with them.
My breasts have gotten so big they make my back and shoulders ache,
Hurt so bad some time, don't know how much more of them I can take.
Wear my bra straps so tight they've left grooves on my skin,
One strap broke; now, I gotta use a big ole safety pin.
Now one breast full of disease, wish it weren't a part of me,
My breasts are now my enemy, and I just want of them to be free.
Got problems with closeness and intimacy, uncomfortable when I'm touched,
That inverted nipple I once hated, wouldn't bother me so much.
I stare in the mirror unable to recognize the body
That stands before me, wounded, scarred, and mutilated.
Gone are the breasts, and the body that I once celebrated.
Breast cancer will make you lose yourself,
Falling deep in despair, sinking in fear, guilt, and shame,
Desperately searching for something, anybody, myself I sometimes blame.
It's not my breasts that make me beautiful, strong, sexy or wise,
Breast are just breasts, they're not the ultimate prize.
Convince all women of this, and maybe then we'll understand,
Beauty's got nothing to do with breasts; they don't go hand in hand.
Live with one or die with two, a choice I shouldn't have to make,
My life I refuse to sacrifice, just for my breasts' sake.

By M. Nicole Bryant

Early Diagnosis and Treatment Can Save Your Life

7
Beyond The Shadows

My three-month check-up went well—another milestone reached. Three months wasn't long in terms of time; however, it was significant for me. Every day, every month that I remained healthy was a good day—I had lived to see another one. I was happy I was making strides in my recovery. I was especially excited that I could resume more physical activity. While I was enjoying my limited exercise regime, I was glad that most of my restrictions were being lifted.

Months passed. I became involved in breast cancer awareness and advocacy. I joined several speakers' bureaus and started publicly discussing my disease. I began to meet more and more women who were breast cancer survivors. I met so many women whose diagnosis was worse and whose treatments were far more serious than mine. My days, and most evenings, were full. Being busy was the best thing that could have happened to me. I didn't have much time to feel sorry for myself. It was still very early in terms of my recovery and survival, and even though I prayed every night, I still needed some kind of sign that would make me feel secure about my future.

This one particular cool and breezy morning I was feeling pretty good. I showered, got dressed and was out the house a little earlier than usual. By the time I arrived at Lake Merritt, my favorite song, "Hero," by Mariah Carey, was blasting through the headset:

And when a hero comes along, with the strength to carry on,
And you cast your fears aside and you know you can survive;
So when you feel like hope is gone, look inside you and be
strong, and you'll finally see the truth that the hero lies in you.

Every single day since I had been home from the hospital I listened to that song. The lyrics echoed so much of what I tried to be: courageous, strong, determined, confident, and self-reliant. As I walked down my usual path, tears streaming down my face, I suddenly noticed the sunlight onto the lake was different than it had ever been. I looked up

Early Diagnosis and Treatment Can Save Your Life

towards the sky. The sky was the bluest of blues with the clouds resembling huge white plumes of smoke. A long ray of sunlight cascaded from the sky onto the lake like a bright reflecting mirror. The rays twinkled on the water, glistening more brightly with every movement. I paused briefly.

Despite the song being loud, I could actually hear other sounds over the music. I removed the earphone from one ear. I looked across the lake at a grove of trees. The leaves danced to their own symphony, almost in time to the music and the wind.

Usually there were three or four sculls on the lake. On this particular morning, there was only one. I could hear the water moving with every row of the paddles. The rowers were in perfect rhythm, back and forth, hypnotizing. The oars moved through the water as if they were gliding through the air. I took my headset completely off my ears, mesmerized by the sounds.

I was convinced things couldn't get any stranger, when suddenly, along came a family of ducks paddling through the water. There were about six of them. I assumed the larger one was the mother. Five little ducks, each smaller than the one in front of it, trailed. I stood there in total disbelief as I watched the family of ducks disappear, one at a time as if they were passing through some sort of portal. Everything was happening in slow motion. It was bizarre and incredible at the same time. I didn't know if I was losing my mind or if I was being prepared to meet my maker. I didn't know quite what it meant, but I knew it meant something.

When I arrived at work, Dena was already there. I said good morning and quietly sat at my desk, reflecting on all the events that had just occurred. I was apprehensive about sharing my morning's experience with her, but I could not keep this to myself. I reluctantly began to tell what had happened.

"Dena, you won't believe what happened to me this morning. The way I look at it, one of two things is happening. I'm either losing my mind or the Good Lord is calling me home."

I began to describe in great detail everything that had occurred. Dena sat at her desk quietly listening to my every word. Then she spoke.

"Well, Nicole, that's one way to look at it, but did you ever think

Early Diagnosis and Treatment Can Save Your Life

those things could be God's way of showing you that this is the beginning of your new life?"

I sat in silence, pondering Dena's wisdom. It never occurred to me that this was a possibility. It didn't dawn on me until then that this experience represented my old life of fear washing away and a new, empowered, cancer-free life drifting ashore.

For so long I had been praying and asking God for any kind of sign to let me know I would be okay, anything that would reassure me He'd heard my prayers. He woke me every day for the past six months; yet, it wasn't enough for me to believe He would spare my life. I couldn't completely separate myself from the shadow of death that the cancer seemed to cast over me. I was just so afraid of dying from the disease I would not allow myself to think I could possibly live a long life; that I could be a survivor. Always in the back of my mind was the five-year survival period. I was nowhere near that anniversary. Most everything I'd done prior to my surgery had been in preparation for my death—not for life. I wondered if the events were my epiphany…I accepted they were.

First, I wanted to lose some unwanted pounds. In addition to the walking, every night for about a week I exercised vigorously, concentrating mostly on an exercise that targeted my waistline. I straddled the chair, placed a stick around my shoulder and proceeded to do one hundred repetitions.

Several days later while taking a shower, an incredibly sharp pain pierced the left side of my chest. Each time I took a breath, the pain increased. I tried to get out of the shower, but couldn't. My sister Angie, who was visiting, had to assist me. I gingerly put on my clothes and then called 911. As I waited for the ambulance to arrive, Angie called my sister Dorothy and told her that I was having a heart attack. Dorothy tried to reassure me I would be okay and should just try to remain calm.

The fire department arrived first. When the paramedics entered the house, I was sitting on the sofa, barely able to move. I described the severe chest pains. One of them quickly hooked me up to a portable EKG monitor. I sat there motionless as the paramedic checked my vital signs.

Early Diagnosis and Treatment Can Save Your Life

"Miss Bryant, I don't know what you're having, but it's definitely not a heart attack. Your heart is strong and there's no indication your heart is under any stress," the medic stated.

I was glad to hear I wasn't having a heart attack. Because the medic couldn't say specifically what was wrong, I was taken to Kaiser Hospital. While I was lying on the gurney in the emergency room, Dr. George walked by.

"Nicole, what are you doing here?" she asked.

"I thought I was having a heart attack, but it was a false alarm."

She took over the examination.

"What have you been doing?" she asked skeptically.

"I've been exercising a little bit."

When I explained to her the type of exercises and that I'd also been moving some furniture around, she scolded me pretty good. Dr. George ordered a chest x-ray and gave me a stern, but sympathetic lecture.

"I certainly want you to continue to exercise, but one hundred of anything is too much right now. Ten is a much better number to start with. Although you might feel you are physically able to do a lot, your body is going to take a long time to heal. Remember, you've had major surgery. You should not lift or push anything heavier than a fork or your TV remote."

She prescribed some medication for the pain and recommended I take the remainder of the day off. I'd learned my lesson. From that day, I was very careful not to do anything that would cause another setback in my recovery.

May brought my six-month check-up with Dr. George, and as with the previous post-surgery visits, everything was fine. Prior to my visit, I'd gathered some information about breast reconstruction. So, I talked to her about the procedure. She recommended I wait at least a year before having the surgery. I was disappointed, but I didn't object. She hadn't given any bad advice to that point, so I decided to wait without question.

A lot of changes were happening in my life during that time as well. I moved from the house that I occupied with Michelle, my granddaughter, and my nephews into an apartment near Lake Merritt. Michelle and

Early Diagnosis and Treatment Can Save Your Life

Briannah moved to Sacramento. The situation at home with my two grown nephews had become increasingly stressful. While I was in the hospital, I agreed to allow them to move into my house. We didn't quite see eye to eye on a lot of things, especially my belief that if I could get up and go to work given my situation, every able-body in the house had to get up also. My morning declaration had become "Get up and do something productive with your life today, because you're not promised tomorrow." They didn't agree with that notion. So, I decided this was a great time to part ways.

    I could not have asked for a better location. The apartment was closer to my job than where I previously lived. I could still walk to and from work, and the area was full of quaint little novelty shops, a theatre, boutiques, Chinese food restaurants, and a grocery store. Everything I needed was within a few blocks.

    This was a whole new beginning for me. For the first time in a very long time, I was going to put my needs first—that it was okay to be selfish. I'd made so many sacrifices for others it was time to do something just for me. Breast cancer made me realize more than ever that the quality of one's life is just as important as quantity.

    Some months later, my relationship with Nathan ended. As kind and giving as he was, Nathan came with some baggage. That's not to say that I didn't have some issues too; however, he had more baggage than I was willing to handle at that point in my life. It seemed like the stronger I got, the further apart we grew. I recognized Nathan needed me more than I needed him. I was still fragile, both physically and emotionally, and wasn't strong enough to take care of him and me too. I also realized our relationship was a lot of work. My health and emotional well-being were far more important than trying to fix a broken relationship. I decided it was okay to be selfish, to put my needs first. In some ways, I think he knew our relationship had run its course. I graciously ended it.

    As time passed, I grew increasingly tired of wearing Mary Jane. It required almost as much care as my real breast. I washed her each night upon removal and placed it in its original box. To lessen the feel of the cold rubbery material next to my body, I placed a piece of tissue

Early Diagnosis and Treatment Can Save Your Life

between my body and it. I had cornered the market on Kleenex. (I refused to buy those special mastectomy bras.) It was awkward when I had to take my bra off at the doctor's office. I never seemed to know where to put Mary Jane—on the chair, on the counter, or hidden under my clothes. Where I placed it really didn't matter to anyone, but I just felt very uncomfortable with it. Mary Jane had intruded on my most intimate moments. I was sick to death of her!

During my nine-month visit with Dr. George, she provided me the name of the plastic surgeon on staff at Kaiser Hospital. I was excited about reaching this point in my recovery, and was thrilled about having the plastic surgery. I was about to embark on another chapter of this saga. I was certain having something more permanent on my chest would alleviate some of my anxieties and insecurities about my body. I was glad to be nearing the date when I could give Mary Jane a final resting place.

While I waited for that day to approach, I couldn't help but reflect on the past year. Oftentimes I was torn between what I knew was important and what society told me was important. I couldn't help but wonder how things would have been if I had decided not to have the mastectomy. Would the lumpectomy have been worse? Would having half a breast been better than having no breast at all? Making peace with my decision was harder than even I anticipated.

I often lamented over why women have to go through this type of mutilation. Men got testicular and prostate cancer all the time. Even in the rare case of penile cancer, men would rather die first than have it cut off. It just didn't seem fair.

Just when I thought I had gotten all my emotions under control, some of those old feelings of self-doubt invaded my thoughts. Outwardly I appeared to have it all together, adjusting very quickly and quite well to my new chest. Inwardly, silently—when I undressed, when I bathed, during intimacy—I felt inadequate, disfigured…ugly. I cried a lot of nights over my loss, not even concerned about whether I would live or die, just wanting my breast back.

From time to time, I would doubt my decision; however, I knew there was really no debate when it came to my breast or my life. I did what I thought was best for me at the time. I did what I thought would give me

Early Diagnosis and Treatment Can Save Your Life

a better chance of living. Nevertheless, the shadow of doubt lingered.

When I was younger, I prayed for everything I thought I wanted—cars, clothes, money, job, a good man, nice house, and oh yes, perfect breasts. Now, even though I prayed for what I knew was important—good health; I still wanted more. I wanted to feel whole.

Satan has a way of getting real busy when you're vulnerable and wounded. He will make you dislike yourself, make you do things you wouldn't normally do, and even make you doubt your faith. But faith was all I had to hold on to until this shadow no longer hovered over me.

Early Diagnosis and Treatment Can Save Your Life

> *Knowing this, that the trying of your faith worketh patience. But let patience have her perfect work, that ye may be perfect and entire, wanting nothing.*
>
> **James 1:3**

Early Diagnosis and Treatment Can Save Your Life

8

Whose Breasts Are These Anyway?

After harboring my share of breast and body issues, I still foolishly thought two breasts would alleviate them. It was getting closer to the day when I could put Mary Jane back into the box in which she came. Like most women, my breasts symbolized my womanhood, but lately, I just wanted them because they were a part of my body. God gave me two of them and that's how I wanted it to be, even if one of them was reconstructed. I knew it did not validate me as a woman; however, I wanted to have a breast back in the spot where one once was.

Everywhere I went—the gym, grocery store, at work, while shopping, walking the lake—I studied other women's breasts, visualizing what mine would eventually look like. I became envious of every woman who had two. While the prosthesis gave me a false sense of security, I couldn't wait to feel natural again. I knew that I wasn't going to be one of those courageous women who after a mastectomy decided to live with one breast. I knew I could never adjust to having just one.

I encountered other women who struggled with the same problem. Several women told me that they never took their clothes off in front of their husbands. I could certainly empathize with them. There were times when I didn't want mine seen or touched either. I also met a woman who had a bilateral mastectomy (both breasts removed). She decided not to have reconstruction. While I admired her taking this stance, I couldn't do it. But believe me, losing a breast, any body part for that matter, is traumatic regardless of how balanced and well adjusted you are (or think you are, as was in my case).

Even though I didn't know anything about either surgery, I was more concerned about what my breasts would like rather than learning the intricacies of the operations. I felt the reconstruction of my left breast was much more important than the reduction of my right one. My left breast had to be reconstructed; reshaped, redefined…it had to be given life again. I figured the breast reduction would be fairly simple

Early Diagnosis and Treatment Can Save Your Life

since the breast was already there. All the surgeon had to do was reduce it to match the size of the reconstructed one. I was giddy with excitement. I could now think about wearing sexy clothes again. I realized I hadn't worn a swimming suit in years. I would finally be able to buy a really pretty bra and panty set. I could finally undress without feeling insecure about my body.

My first visit with Dr. Wagner, the plastic surgeon who would perform the reconstruction and reduction surgeries, was long. Dr. Wagner was on staff at Kaiser Hospital and was recommended to me by Dr. George. Like Dr. George, she was very personable and likeable. She seemed to be quite knowledgeable about both procedures, as she had been practicing for more than twenty years. I was so impressed and so excited that I didn't bother to ask one question.

During the examination, Dr. Wagner discussed my options—implant or the "TRAM" (Transverse Rectus Abdominous Muscle) flap surgery. She carefully explained what to expect, complications, risks, along with the pros and cons of each surgery. I also had to decide if I wanted to go with the saline implant (salt water) or the silicon gel implant which feels more like breast tissue. (I remember when Nurse Bobby from General Hospital got her new silicone gel implants.) At the time, a lot of controversy surrounded the safety of the silicone gel implants, so I wasn't too thrilled about putting a potentially dangerous substance in my already compromised system.

The TRAM flap, on the other hand, was even more appealing because in addition to getting a breast more like my natural one, I could get a tummy tuck to boot—two procedures for the price of one! I was actually leaning more towards the TRAM flap because of this added benefit.

When I discussed the procedure with family and friends, all of my female friends were willing to donate some fat from their bodies just in case I didn't have enough of my own. My sister, Dorothy, convinced me to ask the doctor if she would be a good fat donor candidate. Dr. Wagner informed me while it was possible to use fat from someone else; however, as with any type of transplant, I ran the risk of rejecting her tissue. So, I decided against using her fat. And besides, it wasn't as if I need-

Early Diagnosis and Treatment Can Save Your Life

ed anyone else's, I certainly had plenty of my own to go around.

Unlike the implant surgery, the TRAM flap procedure had several troublesome downsides. I was very uncomfortable with the length of the surgery (at least seven hours) and the complexity of the surgery (tissue is taken from the abdomen and tunneled or surgically transplanted to the new breast site). In addition, the recovery time was months as opposed to weeks with the implant, and the potential complications were far more serious. Also, I did not like the fact I'd be left with another very large scar on my body—one that would literally stretch from hip to hip. Even in this situation, vanity emerged. It may have played an unconscious part in my decision. While there were risks with both surgeries, the risks from the TRAM procedure far exceeded those of the implant surgery. The thought of having a flat stomach was very tempting, but I really wanted something quick and easy. I decided to have the saline implant procedure.

The first phase of my breast reconstruction, the tissue expansion, began in December 1995. This procedure involved inserting a balloon expander beneath my skin and chest muscle. Through a tiny valve mechanism, a salt water solution is periodically injected to gradually fill the expander. Over the course of the next three months, I received weekly injections. It was both fascinating and intriguing as my skin rose from a flattened and disfigured surgery site to a facsimile of a breast. With each visit, my skin stretched until finally, it was time to have the implant inserted.

Naively, I thought when I came home from the hospital with my two new and what I called 'functional breasts,' I would be transformed into a whole woman again. Nothing could have been further from the truth.

My surgery was scheduled for April 24, 1996. I proceeded to the eighth floor where I registered. A short time later, a nurse came to inform me that Dr. Wagner had been delayed with another surgery. While I patiently waited, I watched the soaps—<u>Young and The Restless</u> (11:00 a.m.), <u>All My Children</u> (12:00 p.m.), <u>One Life To Live</u> (1:00 p.m.). Not much had changed since the last time I watched them when I was in the hospital. About halfway through <u>One Life To Live</u>, the

Early Diagnosis and Treatment Can Save Your Life

nurse came back into the room.

"Ms. Bryant, we're ready for you."

"Finally," I whispered.

I was wheeled to the fifth floor surgery waiting area, only a few feet from the elevator door. As the door opened and closed, I could see other patients as they were being wheeled in and out of the surgery area. Several doctors walked by, removing their surgery head garments as they passed.

The wait seemed like a long time, but it was only about ten minutes or so. The elevator door opened, and Dr. Wagner exited. As she came closer, I noticed a purple magic marker nestled between her fingers and a tape measure around her neck. After apologizing for being late, she escorted me into a smaller room where she took another set of measurements. I watched intently as she placed x's, o's and other identifying marks on both sides of my chest.

"What size would you like the right breast to be, Nicole?" she asked as she continued to map the dimensions of my new breasts.

"A 36C, a nice handful," I answered enthusiastically.

"Then a 36C it is," she responded.

Once the measurements were complete, I was taken back to the waiting area. Five minutes later the gurney arrived and I was wheeled into the operating room. I instantly reverted to my prior surgery. As I lay there staring at the ceiling into the large overhead light, I said one last prayer.

"God please guide the surgeon's hands. Watch over and keep me. Let Your will be done, Amen"

The anesthesiologist prepped me. When the IV was inserted in my hand, I was reminded of how much I hated this part of the procedure. He inserted the sedative into the needle. I could feel the coolness of the medicine circulating through my veins. It took effect very quickly.

"Ms. Bryant, do you know what surgery you're having today?" she asked.

"Yes, you're going to give me a new…"

I felt myself getting drowsy. My eyelids became heavy, everything was out of focus, and my body completely relaxed. I don't even think I

Early Diagnosis and Treatment Can Save Your Life

completed my response.

It seemed like the surgery had only taken a few minutes; however, it actually lasted more than two hours. When I awoke, I cried uncontrollably. Dr. Wagner was sitting by my bedside. I could hear her instruct the recovery room nurse to bring me something for my pain. Funny thing though, I was hurting, but it wasn't physical. It was far deeper and more intense than what I'd ever experienced from physical pain. I was inconsolable.

I was transferred me to a private room. Michelle and Dorothy stopped to visit but didn't stay long. I remained groggy from the anesthesia and was in and out of sleep most of the time. Each time I awoke, I felt more disconnected than previously. I couldn't seem to shake the despondency.

The nurse periodically checked on me. I thought if I'd just give myself another shot of the morphine that I wouldn't have to deal with what I was feeling. I fell asleep briefly, but woke up again feeling the same. Taking more medication couldn't comfort me.

Later that night while lying quietly in bed, I suddenly remembered. I tried to sit up, but I couldn't.

"I remember," I cried in a deep whisper.

Instantly, it all came back and I knew why I felt so sad, why I felt so much anguish. I was fully awake and I wasn't dreaming. Some experts call it an out-of-body experience; others believe that people who have similar experiences are in a deep dream state. I'm not sure what it was, or what to call it, but I do know that something happened to me that day in the operating room.

I recalled hearing the anesthesiologist ask me if I knew what surgery I was having.

I awoke to this tremendously bright, almost blinding, light. It encompassed the entire space. It was magnificently brilliant. I floated off the gurney. Off in the distance, I could see a figure coming closer to me. Initially, I couldn't make out who or what it was, but as the figure drew closer, I recognized her. It was my best friend, Jo. Dressed in this long white robe, only her face and hands were visible. The closer she came towards me, the more lifelike she seemed. She was beautiful and

Early Diagnosis and Treatment Can Save Your Life

ageless.

"Oh, Jo," I cried. "I'm so glad to see you; I've missed you so much."

"I know, Nikki," she said softly.

"I want to come with you, Jo."

I reached out my hand to touch her. A very peaceful, angelic expression captivated her face. She gently put my hand into hers and in a soft vibrating whisper said,

"You can't come with me right now, Nikki."

"But I want to," I cried.

She released my hand, clasped her hands into each other and spoke the same words again to me, but firmer this time.

"No, not now, you can't come with me."

Then she slowly faded away.

The next thing I remember was waking up to Dr. Wagner sitting by my bed in the recovery room. To this day, I have not been able to describe how terribly sad I was that she wouldn't let me go with her. I now understood why I was crying when I awoke from the surgery. I'd cried so much since being diagnosed that I didn't think I had any more tears to shed. I've often heard tears make you strong, but I wasn't feeling it. I felt vulnerable, abandoned, and I was grieving, but more than anything, I was ready to be with my friend and with God. I knew she was in heaven because it was beautiful. It would have been okay with me if I'd died.

Dr. Wagner came to see me the next day. Everything seemed to be healing properly. I told her about my "out-of-body-experience." She said it gave her chills, and that she understood why I was crying. This surgery wasn't nearly physically draining as it was emotionally grueling.

My stay in the hospital was relatively short compared to when I had the mastectomy. Only three days this time. I spent most of the last two days in the hospital thinking about Jo and my experience at the lake. I knew the two were somehow connected.

The night before I left the hospital I didn't get any sleep. I prayed to God to help me understand. When I awoke the next morning, I felt as if the weight of the world had been lifted. For the first time since that Friday afternoon when I was told I had breast cancer, I wasn't worried about dying from it. Through my friend, God had shown me He wasn't ready for me yet. He was going to keep me here to do His will. I didn't know why and wasn't going to question it. It's amazing how He works.

I was eager to experience my new breasts. Just having a mound on both sides of my chest felt good again. Little did I know of the unforeseen challenges. Unlike the mastectomy, where only one side of my body was affected, both sides of my body were cut on, cut up, and cut out. The swelling was more noticeable. My first night home was pretty miserable. As the days and nights passed, it got progressively worse.

The discomfort increased over the next several days. I couldn't lie down, couldn't get up, and couldn't use either arm. I was miserable. Going to the bathroom was especially challenging. (Try going to the bathroom and not use your arms and you'll understand what I mean.)

I had been home three days and hadn't slept a full night. By now, the swelling had gotten increasingly worse, intensifying the pain. The swelling was so pronounced I had to hold both my arms up and away from my body like a scarecrow. Any amount of movement hurt. I was pitiful and I was mad. I hadn't even considered that I would be unable to take care of myself; nor had I counted on the recovery being quite this difficult. Foolishly, I thought once I had the surgery, I could just put on a bra and be done with it.

I finally called George and asked him if he could come and take care of me. I suppose I could have called one of my girlfriends or family, but I didn't. George had a lot of patience and I knew that patience was going to be needed for this task.

The first night he slept in the bed with me. Neither one of us got much sleep. Each time I had to get up, he had to get up to help me get out of bed. The next morning, we knew we had to figure out where each of us was going to sleep because the bed wasn't going to work—not with us both in it at the same time.

Finally, we figured it out. George brought the recliner/rocker from the living room into the bedroom. He rearranged the bed so I would have enough room to maneuver around the chair and the bed without

Early Diagnosis and Treatment Can Save Your Life

bumping into things. He put four pillows on each side to cushion my arms, and several more were used for my head rest. That recliner became my bed for the next twelve days. The chair reclined far enough so that my body was fully extended. When I needed to get out of the chair, I would use the lever to bring me back to a sitting position. All I had to do was use the strength from my legs to pull myself out of the chair. Had it not been for that recliner, I don't know if George and I would have remained friends. I wasn't the easiest person to get along with then. Thank God for that recliner, and thank God for George.

I had my check-up with Dr. Wagner, and according to her, I was healing well. She removed the original bandages and replaced them with new ones. The swelling had gone down somewhat and I was regaining some mobility in my arms.

I finally started feeling like a human being again. I was also becoming increasingly more curious and excited about seeing my new breasts.

One morning while George was out, I decided I wanted to see what my new breasts looked like. I gingerly walked into the bathroom, turned on all the lights and removed the bandages from both incisions. I couldn't believe what I saw.

Shock cascaded into tears. Stitches were everywhere. The scar on my right breast stretched from my inner chest to nearly half way around my back. My new, reconstructed breast didn't look anything like a breast. It looked more like half a grapefruit resting on my chest. It was round, with no contour at all. It had no nipple or areola (which I knew would be applied later). The mastectomy incision was noticeably visible, separating the grapefruit-shaped mound on my chest in half. This scar also seemed longer than necessary. It stretched from the inside of the left side of my chest to under my left arm. I cried even more than when my breast was removed.

I composed myself long enough to call my girlfriend, Marsha. When she answered the phone, I was still crying. Before she could say hello, I babbled hysterically,

"Marsha, this doctor has f...ed me up. I'm more disfigured now than I was when they removed my breast. They cut me from pillar to post. My chest looks like a barbed wire fence. Bandages and scars are

Early Diagnosis and Treatment Can Save Your Life

everywhere. My right breast is so lopsided that it's almost under my arm. There is a big hole under my right breast that's still bleeding. The areola is all the same size as it was when I was a 40D. There's more areola than breast. My left side is as hard as a brick and it's shaped funny. It doesn't even look like a breast. And to make matters worse, I haven't had a good night's sleep in about twelve days. I swear, if my breasts don't start falling into place or looking any better in a few days, I'm going to start looking for an attorney and sue this damn doctor."

I got this entire spiel out without taking a breath. I was mad as hell.

"Girl, what is wrong with your crazy ass? Take a breath before you fall out or something," she said jokingly.

"Marsha, you wouldn't believe this shit. My chest is f...ed up. I look an absolute mess and I'm mad as hell. My breasts don't look anything like my Reach to Recovery volunteer's."

Marsha broke out in laughter, which made me laugh also. My hysteria was gone and I was able speak more calmly.

"I'm so pissed. I thought the reconstruction and reduction was going to make my breasts better. Instead it made it worse."

"When do you go back to see the doctor?" she asked.

"I just had my appointment. I took the bandages off because I wanted to see what they looked like."

"That's what your ass gets for being so nosy."

If anyone could make me see the humor in this situation, Marsha could. Although I wasn't looking for any, I needed it. I really appreciated her because she could always find something funny to say in the most difficult of situations. She tried to convince me once everything healed my breasts would look better. I wasn't so convinced.

When I finished talking to Marsha, I called my Reach To Recovery Volunteer. Jackie wasn't available when I called, but she returned my call later that day. By the time she did, I was able to articulate more calmly what my concerns were. When I told her about all the scars, she was quick to remind me that she had some also. I didn't recall seeing scars on her, particularly this many. She tried to assure me her scars were visible as well. I asked her if she could come over and let me see her breasts again.

Early Diagnosis and Treatment Can Save Your Life

Jackie came over the very next day. I quickly ushered her into my living room, sat her on the sofa and with her permission, started to re-inspect her breasts. On her very first visit after my mastectomy, I was so impressed with her breast reconstruction. As I examined every inch of them, I noticed this time that she did have a few scars, but they weren't nearly as pronounced as mine. Her reconstructed breast looked more natural. Jackie tried to convince me that once the swelling went down, after the incisions healed, and when gravity did its thing, my breasts would look better and I would feel better about the results. She left me a tape about reconstruction and reduction surgery and suggested I watch it.

I'm embarrassed to admit that prior to the reconstruction surgery I didn't bother to do my homework. I didn't check Dr. Wagner's credentials. I didn't check to see how many of these surgeries she had performed. I didn't ask to see before and after pictures of her work. I didn't do anything. Because she worked at the hospital, was recommended by Dr. George, and coupled with my desperation to regain some of my self-esteem, I relinquished what good judgment I had. Once she explained the pros and cons of each surgery, I was sold. I just assumed she would do a good job. I would have my breasts and everything would be right with the world and me. It didn't happen.

Once again my breasts tormented me. It wasn't supposed to turn out like this. The next day, I was depressed all over again. Certainly God didn't spare me just to go through this. When I was diagnosed with breast cancer, I never once asked God why me. But now, I questioned why He spared me. If there was a lesson to be had, I didn't have a clue.

I wanted the implant out of my chest. The more I thought about it, the angrier I got. How could any doctor think anyone would want her chest looking like mine? I stayed pissed for a couple of days, then got the Yellow Pages and called at least six different plastic surgeons that specialized in breast reduction and reconstruction surgery. I requested information from each one of them and anxiously waited for the material to arrive.

I received the first pamphlet about two days later. When I compared my surgery with the pictures in the pamphlet, I was even madder. Over

Early Diagnosis and Treatment Can Save Your Life

the next several days, brochures arrived from each of the other doctors. When I finished looking at them, I was beyond mad. None of the pictures in any of the six brochures remotely resembled what mine looked like.

Both of my breasts were ugly and I hated them all over again. It was bad enough that I had to lose a breast to cancer, but now my good one was messed up. The incision on my right breast should have been curved more like a half moon, under the fold of the breast. Instead, the incision was straight across my chest which caused my breast to lean outward towards my arm.

I spent days thinking about what my chest would have looked like if I'd had the TRAM surgery. I figured it couldn't have been any worse, in spite of the risks. I began to wonder if Dr. Wagner actually performed the surgery since it didn't look like the work of an experienced surgeon. I wondered if that young doctor who I'd met in her office on a previous visit and who was in the operating room during my procedure had actually performed it. The longer I looked at the pictures, the angrier I became at Dr. Wagner. I wasn't looking for perfection; I knew that was only God's to give. I did, however, expect to get a better job than what I'd gotten. I also began to blame myself for not taking a more active role in deciding which procedure would have been best for me.

I was feeling overwhelmed by my disfigured chest, second-guessing my decision, wishing I had opted for the other procedure. Maybe I would have been better off without the reconstruction and reduction. This procedure was supposed to make me feel whole and happy again; instead it left me feeling depressed and looking more disfigured than when I had just one breast.

One would think given all my blessings, I wouldn't question anything that happened in my life, but I did. Sometimes our emotions are beyond our control, particularly when we're vulnerable. I had to look at my body every day for the rest of my life. I should at the least, like the reflection.

While recuperating, I learned one of my first cousins was diagnosed with breast cancer and wasn't doing well. With a lot of prayer, I was able to put things in perspective. Surprisingly, as my wounds slowly healed, I became less angry at Dr. Wagner and more thankful I was alive. I also stopped being angry at myself. This didn't mean I was feel-

Early Diagnosis and Treatment Can Save Your Life

ing warm and fuzzy, but learning of my cousin's situation made me realize how blessed I was. There were far more important things in life than my breasts—my overall health was the most important thing. I could get new breasts if I wanted them. I couldn't, on the other hand, get another life. Besides, better breasts wouldn't do me a bit of good if the cancer came back.

I kept my follow-up appointment with Dr. Wagner. During a long discussion, I was able to articulate my feelings and concerns to her without being angry or critical. Dr. Wagner told me it was common to be overwhelmed by the initial appearance of the plastic surgery. She reassured me that once the implant 'settled' in place, it would look better. And, once the refinement surgeries (areola and nipple reconstruction) were complete, my breast would look more natural and I would feel better about the outcome. We didn't discuss my right breast at all. I had spent so much time in the last months thinking and talking about my breasts, I was almost tired of them.

Unlike with the mastectomy where I returned to work immediately, I took nearly six weeks off with this surgery. I'd earned a lot of comp time so I used all the hours to recuperate.

When I returned to work, my co-workers were both fascinated and curious about my new breasts. One of them, Jacqueline, had a new question for me every day. She even wanted to see how the implant looked and what it felt like. I allowed her to feel it. She asked me about everything from how I felt when I first made love after my mastectomy to if I was scared of dying from the breast cancer. I was very candid with her. I think we both learned a lot that summer. Her questions helped me to deal with a lot of stuff I hadn't shared with anyone. Our conversations were both therapeutic and enlightening.

My granddaughters, on the other hand, remained quite awestruck with them. Before the reconstruction they would ask me, "NaNa, when are you going to get your new titty?" Now it was, "NaNa, when are you going to get your new nipple?" I think they were confused by how my body went from having two breasts, then one breast, then back to two.

I remembered how they watched me as I removed Mary Jane from my bra. They stared with curiosity and amazement, focusing on the side

Early Diagnosis and Treatment Can Save Your Life

of my chest where my left breast once was. Their stares were now of puzzlement. Even though at the time of my diagnosis they were very young, Briannah was five and Jerica was four, I still talked to them about breast cancer. They didn't have a clue about the seriousness of my condition. I never let them see me cry, nor did I allow them to think that I would die. If it hadn't been for them, I would have given up.

Inasmuch as I tried not to dwell on my breasts, it was hard to do. It wasn't as if I couldn't notice them. My dislike for both the reconstruction and reduction was equally shared. I was more uncomfortable with my body after the plastic surgery than I was following the mastectomy. The reconstructed one particularly bothered me. I'd hoped that the implant would take on the shape and contour of a breast. It didn't. I even hoped that it would sag a bit. It never did. As a matter of fact, the implant seemed to become harder instead of softer.

My right breast appeared to be leaning more towards my right arm and the scars that ran across my chest were quite visible. Despite being unhappy with the way they looked, on two different occasions I cancelled the refinement surgery. I wasn't sure if I wanted Dr. Wagner to operate on me again. So I made appointments to see several other plastic surgeons in the area.

One of them was a member of the team of doctors that examined me at Alta Bates Hospital. When I met with the plastic surgeon, I asked to see before and after photos, and asked a lot more questions this time. I was impressed with his work until he said he thought the surgeon had done a pretty good job on me. There was no way that anyone could think this was a good job. Because of that, I decided not to use him.

I also made an appointment with the plastic surgeon that performed Jackie's reconstruction. However, by the time I was supposed to see this doctor, I decided to just forget it. Having the refinement surgeries didn't seem all that important any more. There was very little I could do about how my breasts turned out. I could, on the other hand, be in total control of how I turned out. My breasts had consumed enough of my time, my thoughts, and my energy.

Months turned into years, and before I knew it, I was celebrating my three-year anniversary. I was a survivor!

Early Diagnosis and Treatment Can Save Your Life

The isolation I once felt no longer existed. I was very active in breast cancer awareness and advocacy, speaking at churches, community organizations, colleges, a women's prison, several support groups, participating in forums, workshops, focus groups and a TV segment on breast cancer. The more I helped others, the more my purpose was revealed. I had become comfortable in my role as an educator and activist. I'd learned so much during the past years about staying emotionally, physically, and spiritually healthy. A better me emerged out of this living hell.

And while I was willing to give up some things, I wasn't willing to give up everything. I'd heard catfish retained toxins in its fatty tissue longer than most other fish and because it was a scavenger we shouldn't eat it anyway. Well, I figured I'd already given up so much already. I'd given up my breast, I'd given up sex, and I'd given up some bad habits. I wasn't about to give up my fried catfish. I had to draw a line somewhere. I tried acupuncture instead.

One event had such a profound effect on me that it completely changed my attitude about my breasts and my life. In October 1997, I participated in a three-day retreat sponsored by the Charlotte Maxwell Complementary Clinic (CMCC). CMCC provided alternative therapies and services for low-income women with cancer. Nearly fifty-five breast cancer survivors attended.

There were women of all races, shapes and sizes; young women and old women, women with disabilities, professional and non-professional, women in different stages of their breast cancer diagnoses. Women with hair. Some were bald. Some wore scarves, and others wore wigs. Some had endured several bouts with breast cancer; others were recently diagnosed. Some were recovering from chemotherapy and radiation, while others were battling both breast and cervical cancers.

Of all the women who attended the retreat, there was one young lady who particularly touched not only me, but most of the women there. I'll call her Maria.

Maria was a very soft-spoken Hispanic woman who, through her interpreter, said that she had been diagnosed with breast cancer and had undergone a mastectomy and breast reconstruction. She possessed a

Early Diagnosis and Treatment Can Save Your Life

sad, overcast spirit. She didn't smile very much; you could sense something troubling her. She was a small figure of a woman with long black hair and large, expressive brown eyes that appeared to have no life in them.

One day while we were all gathered sharing our personal experiences and praising God, Maria began to cry as she stood up and slowly raised her blouse to show us her scars. Nearly everyone gasped. It was supposed to have been reconstruction; instead, a grossly disfigured mutilation rested upon her chest.

Her chest looked as if a bomb had exploded and a blind surgeon put her back together. Frankenstein stitches zigzagged across her chest, resembling a jig-saw puzzle whose pieces were in the wrong place, but sewn together anyway. You had to see it to believe it. It was hard to imagine a licensed physician, in the United States of America, could have done this to her, but to everyone's shock and disbelief, it was performed at a hospital in Northern California.

I don't know if I could have been as brave as Maria. I don't think I would have wanted to live if my surgery had turned out like hers. I said a prayer for her. We all did. I was overwhelmed to the point of tears and ashamed of myself. I had been complaining because my implant looked funny and that scars were longer than they should have been. I thought I had been disfigured. My scars paled in comparison to hers.

Maria's chest haunted me for months, but a blessing came out of that experience. After seeing Maria, I began to appreciate my body more. Even though my surgery wasn't as good as it could have been, it now seemed insignificant. I realized that things could have been so much worse; and because they weren't, I was extremely grateful. From that day on, I let go of my insecurities and hang ups.

My mother used to say that we should be thankful for what we have because there's always someone out there with a situation that is worse and who would gladly exchange places. I thanked God for what I had, not what I thought I needed. This was the beginning of my spiritual rebirth.

Breast cancer changed me in more ways than I thought imaginable...I finally got it! My breasts were just breasts, a body part. They

Early Diagnosis and Treatment Can Save Your Life

weren't the measure of my beauty; they didn't determine my strength, they didn't control my existence or my destiny; nor did they define me as a woman. My life would go on with or without them. I let go of so many things. I knew I could never change the past, but I could do a lot to change my future.

Early Diagnosis and Treatment Can Save Your Life

And He said unto me: My grace is sufficient for thee; for my strength is made perfect in weakness.

2 Corinthians 12:9

Early Diagnosis and Treatment Can Save Your Life

9

Still On My Journey

In July 2000, I returned home to East Carondelet, Illinois to care for my mother. I really hadn't given much thought to all I was giving up—my family, my job, my doctors, my close friends—essentially my lifelines. I soon discovered that in addition to giving up a lot of things, I was giving up a bit of myself as well. I knew coming back home was going to present some challenges for me, but I was prepared. Breast cancer had been an excellent teacher and I was a very good student. Since I had successfully survived cancer for nearly six years, I wasn't as concerned about my health as I was my mother's. While I knew it was important to stay healthy, I was more than willing to sacrifice my health to take care of her.

When I made plans to move, I neglected to give any thought to relinquishing health coverage. Given all I'd learned and preached to other women, I was still playing Russian Roulette with my health and possibly my life. As I'd done in the past, I was relying on my strength, my faith, and a lot of prayer to get me through this situation.

Taking care of my mother and overseeing the care of my 92 year-old grandmother, who was in a nursing home, took all my time and energy. Not only had I gone more than a year without a mammogram and clinical exam (my last one had been in 1999), but I performed breast self-exams only when I had the energy to do them, which was sporadic at best.

In October 2001, I was able to find a clinic that would give me a mammogram based on my income, which at the time was next to nothing. Because of my history, they referred me to Barnes Breast Cancer Center in St. Louis, Missouri. As in the past, I was very anxious before, during, and after the exam. This time I had cause to be.

Following the clinical exam, I was given a mammogram. To my horror, the mammogram revealed two suspicious spots in my right breast. All the fear and blame came rushing back.

"Not again," I prayed. "Oh God, please don't let this be happening again."

I was immediately scheduled to have an ultrasound. I waited lifeless on the table for the doctor to begin her exam. The doctor, nurse, and ultrasound technician all entered the room. The technician rolled the ultrasound machine on the right side of the bed. The procedure was quick and the results even quicker. The doctor tried to reassure me that the lumps appeared to be nothing more than cysts. I wasn't quite so sure. I tried to remain calm, but the fear was paralyzing. Going through breast cancer once was bad enough. The thought of having to go through it again seemed unbearable.

The doctor performed the aspiration immediately. I watched the screen as she inserted the needle into the lump. It began to deflate as if it were a pricked balloon.

"Just as I suspected," she said triumphantly.

"Now the other one."

She inserted the needle into the second lump. Again, the cyst disappeared from the screen. Tears began to swell.

"Thank you, God. Thank you, thank you, thank you," I whispered.

And just like that, the crisis was over. The doctor patted me on my shoulder.

"It's important that you have a mammogram every year."

"Yes Mam, I know," I said, fighting back the tears. "You won't have to worry about me; I won't miss another one—ever."

When the doctors left the room, I broke down. This scare was far more emotional than the initial diagnosis. I was so sure that since I'd made it past the five-year mark, I didn't have anything to worry about. I was wrong. I have since learned that breast cancer can come back at any time, and for up to thirty years. I got dressed, went home, and my mother never knew; no one did. I turned fifty that December; I received my gift that October.

As I entered my fifties, my breasts still played a lead role in my health. By early 2004, the original implant had gotten worse. It felt like a brick lying on my chest and was causing me some pain. It also appeared to have shifted somewhat. My physician at Barnes referred me to a plastic surgeon. As it turned out, I had seen her in a TV segment

Early Diagnosis and Treatment Can Save Your Life

about breast reconstruction.

I called Dr. Trudeau's office and got an appointment immediately. I arrived at her office excited about the surgery. While sitting on the examining room table waiting for the plastic surgeon to enter, I noticed a picture on the wall. It was of a stone-like female figure resembling Venus de Milo. Both her arms were cut off just below her shoulders, but interestingly enough, she had both her breasts. They were perfectly shaped, nipples saluting at attention. The caption underneath read: ***Service performed to reshape normal structures of the body in order to improve a patient's appearance and self-esteem.***

"Why are you so troubled by the picture's caption?" I questioned myself. *"You're here to do just what the caption said, you're getting a new implant, the nipple constructed, and the areola tattooed on your left breast, all to improve your appearance and self-esteem, to make you feel whole."*

I thought, "It's no wonder we're all confused and messed up about our bodies and images of beauty. Here's a picture of a woman with half a body, no arms, no legs, yet her breasts are perfect." I reconciled that this procedure was a necessity; whereas for others it was optional.

After Dr. Trudeau completed her examination, she explained to me it was common for the implant to need replacement after five or six years. The hardness was probably from scar tissue that had encased the implant. I was glad when she recommended that it be removed. I never really liked the implant—I just learned to live with it.

Not only would the implant be replaced, and the areola and nipple constructed, but my right breast would also be realigned so it wouldn't lean outward so much. I was somewhat uneasy about more plastic surgery, always concerned something would go wrong. However, I knew deep down inside I was ready to get this thing off my chest and replace it with something that resembled a breast. Regardless of the outcome, this was going to be the absolute last time anything was going to be done to them—good, bad, ugly, or indifferent. I would live with it.

The surgery was performed on an outpatient basis with the entire procedure only taking a few hours. According to my doctor it was successful. Since there were no complications and my recovery time much

Early Diagnosis and Treatment Can Save Your Life

quicker than expected, I returned home that evening.

I finally got the nipple on my left breast. Even with all the improvements, I realized that my breasts will never be what they once were; they will never be perfect. I'm in a good place now, and I'm okay with them.

My breasts and I have come full circle. We've been through a lot. One formally housed the disease that could have possibly ended my life. They helped me regain my perspective about inner strength, beauty, and faith. They accommodated my insecurities and ignorance, contributed to my innermost vulnerabilities, served as the foundation to rebuild my self-esteem, and propelled my spiritual rebirth.

Prior to breast cancer, I believed that being sexy was about attitude and had nothing to do with one's physical appearance. Breast cancer changed that. After my diagnosis, I was left feeling inadequate, vulnerable, and emotionally fragile. I allowed myself to believe my womanhood had a direct correlation to my breasts. Funny how your attitude readjusts when something life-altering happens to you. Once the fog lifted, I was able to resolve my breast issues and release the anguish that I'd held for so long. I began a new love affair with life, which meant loving myself even more than I could have ever imagined.

I've discovered that it doesn't matter if you have one breast, two slightly different breasts, or no breasts at all. What is important is that you love yourself enough to not let anything or anyone compromise your health and well-being. I know now it wasn't, nor isn't, my breasts that make me special. Having breast cancer just made me lose sight of that, temporarily.

My breast health will be a part of my life forever; however, I refuse to let them dictate my emotional well-being. I've had a lot of time to heal and for reflection. I'm no longer obsessed with having 'perfect' breasts. I no longer ache for the perky little nipple along with the perfectly sized areola. At one time, I thought having my new symbols of womanhood would make me complete and would resolve all my breasts issues.

Well, ten years after my initial diagnosis, eight years after my first reconstruction, and nearly two years since my last corrective surgery,

Early Diagnosis and Treatment Can Save Your Life

there is *still* a noticeable indentation on my reconstructed breast. The reconstructed breast is *still* slightly higher than the right breast. My right breast is *still* slightly larger than my left breast. The scars *still* stretch across my chest and underarms, and I finally have a nipple on my left breast that isn't inverted. My breasts *still* matter, but for different reasons. They are not the most important things in life, they didn't help make me whole, nor will they help save my soul.

It took losing a part of me to remind myself that physical beauty can be gone in a flash. Inner beauty lasts forever. I have come to terms with the loss of my breast and everything in between, and that having or not having a body part will never make me any less a woman. It's ironic that my emotional enlightenment and transformation was aided by my uninvited and unwanted physical metamorphosis. I'm more woman not because of them, but in spite of them. I'm a better human being because of the journey. I love life so much more than my breasts!

Every day, every minute, every breath is a new beginning and one where I continue to learn things about myself, to understand my limitations, to recognize my strengths, and to not be ashamed of my weaknesses. I now strive for good health, soundness of mind, and spiritual peace. I've also learned that cancer is a life experience—once you've been diagnosed with it, it's a part of your journey forever. It affects every aspect of your existence—your family, your partner, your job, your financial matters, including your outlook on life.

What's even more deceiving about this disease or any potentially life-threatening illness is that it can have a profound affect on your relationship with God. It will test your faith; maybe even make you to lose it. It will have you wondering if prayer makes a difference and doubting everything about His goodness and mercy.

I recognized early in my diagnosis that breast cancer was bigger than me; but not better than me… and certainly no match for God. I could not fight this battle alone so I called on "The One" who I knew would not only fight the battle but win the war.

I've also learned that each day is a priceless gift, an opportunity for God to do something miraculous. Breast cancer allowed me to take a remarkable and awesome journey of personal growth and spiritual heal-

Early Diagnosis and Treatment Can Save Your Life

ing. It took me to my destination of reclaiming my soul and finding my way back to God. Maybe I would have found my way back to Him without breast cancer. I don't know. One thing I know for sure—cancer was the vehicle that got me there sooner. I also know that this was exactly the journey I was supposed to take.

It really hit home that we never know what life has in store for us. There's an old saying that goes "we know where we've been, but we don't always know where we're going." And in my case, for a period of my life, I didn't have a clue which direction it was headed. I'd made some bad choices, wasted a lot of time doing nothing. I hadn't been to church in years and I wasn't giving God any of my time. "God is a jealous God," the scriptures say. I was too busy having too much fun to serve Him or to let Him in my life. I am confident in knowing that anything that God leads me to, He'll lead me through. Breast cancer gave me direction and purpose. I feel very strongly that having this disease was spiritually mandated for my soul's reawakening.

I've always been a child of God, but I'm the first to admit that I haven't always acted like a Christian. I'm so glad that God isn't concerned about where I've been, but where I'm going. Prior to embarking on this life-changing journey, I was spiritually lost. Even then, I had the good sense to always ask Him to forgive me for my sins, and to bless and keep me. I also knew that it was prayer (from my mother and others) that got me through the bad times as well as the good times.

One of my mother's favorite sayings when she faced a crisis was that God doesn't put more on you than you can bear. When I was young, I didn't know what she meant. It wasn't until I became an adult and things happened in my life that made me question my faith, that I understood her words.

After breast cancer, I relied heavily on those things my mother taught me about God's love, faith, and prayer—it works when nothing else does. For a long time I prayed for all the wrong things. Now, I pray for understanding. I pray for strength. I pray for guidance. I pray for healing. More than money, more than breasts, more than any other material thing, my daily prayer is for good health, and that He continues to guide my footsteps.

Early Diagnosis and Treatment Can Save Your Life

I know my life was spared for a reason. I believe one of the reasons was to return home to care for my mother and grandmother. Sadly though, both have passed away. My grandmother died in January 2001. My mother made her transition in September 2004. She was seventy-four. Caring for them was one of those detours I had to take in order to reconnect spiritually and to submit to God's will in my life. I also know that He is not through with me yet!

I believe part of the work I'm supposed to do is to help other people. Telling my story is just one of the ways I'm doing this. I hope that by sharing, I can help alleviate some of the fear, helplessness, and yes, ignorance that is associated with this disease. I was overcome with fear when I was diagnosed. It is a powerful emotion. The stronger the fear, the more vulnerable and helpless one can feel. We fear what we don't understand. In my case, I was scared to death of breast cancer because I knew absolutely nothing about it. Ignorance perpetuates the notion that we are victims. We are victims only if we allow ourselves to be consumed by the despair that follows a breast cancer diagnosis.

There were times when I was haunted by the possibility of knowing that my breasts (or rather a disease of the breasts) could end my life. The thought of a possible reoccurrence was overwhelmingly frightening. Every time I got an ache or pain on the left side of my chest, I just knew the cancer had returned. Now, if I get a pain there, it's just that—a pain.

Time, prayer, and wisdom helped me put my demons to bed. I've refused to live in fear of losing my life to breast cancer. I've had several people ask me if I was afraid of dying from it. I would answer them "No" because I knew that this disease could not defeat Him. I knew that I'd go when God wanted me to go; not when breast cancer said so.

I am aware that I had a disease that is like a sleeping giant. It could rear its ugly head at any time, without notice or consideration of me or my feelings and wreak havoc on my body. But even knowing that it can return doesn't frighten me. I am, on the other hand, sad so many women will lose their lives to this beast. I'm even sadder that so many, many women have to suffer to beat it. I'm mortified that in this day of test tube babies, men on Mars, heart transplants, cloning, sex change oper-

Early Diagnosis and Treatment Can Save Your Life

ations, and other modern-day medical marvels there is still no cure for this destructive ailment. It is at those times I am most thankful to God for blessing me and keeping me healthy. I remind myself that everything happens for a reason and God has a purpose for everything.

Most of us share similar experiences in life. Breast cancer survivors have a common thread creating an unbreakable life-long bond and kinship. Our scars—scars that remind us of the battles we've fought and won, forever connect us. We are a sisterhood of brave, purposeful, and prayerful warriors who will never give in, give up, or give out. We stand together in our unwavering fight to stay healthy; to overcome our insecurities, to regain our sense of self, and to maintain our dignity. We remain steadfast in our faith; resolute in our commitment to educating others and ourselves about this disease. Our survival is a testament to the will of God and to the fact that He will fight our battles.

I'm looking forward to living a long, healthy, and productive life. In December of 2005, I celebrated my fifty-fourth birthday. They say that the fifties are the new forties. I don't know when that happened, but I don't mind getting older anymore. I'm fifty-four, look forty-four, feel thirty-four, and I'm living my life like it's golden because I now know it is. I have embraced the aging process with confidence, pride, and dignity—along with Ms. Clairol. For every year that I get older, I have another opportunity to celebrate life and God's many blessings.

My journey was more than just about this disease. It has been an incredible life-altering, life-affirming, and rewarding voyage. Had it not been for breast cancer, I never would have learned to really appreciate my imperfections. Had it not been for breast cancer, I never would have learned to be happy (and thankful) for what God has given me. Had it not been for breast cancer, I would not have learned to rejoice in the magnificence of how He created me. Had it not been for breast cancer, I would not have experienced the Divine Providence of God in my life.

Sometimes you have to go through something in order to get somewhere. Breast cancer was my "something." My "somewhere" was being reconnected with God. I accept that breast cancer will be a part of my life for as long as God blesses me with life. I am secure in knowing that God loves me, and that my relationship with Him transcends any dis-

Early Diagnosis and Treatment Can Save Your Life

ease, challenge, or obstacle that confronts me. I pray God will continue to do profound things in my life for I recognize my journey has really just begun. I am on this road for the ultimate prize…my soul's salvation and everlasting life. Until then, I'm still on it.

Early Diagnosis and Treatment Can Save Your Life

> *But they that wait upon the Lord shall renew their strength; they shall mount up with wings as eagles, they shall run, and not be weary; and they shall walk, and not faint.*
>
> **Isaiah 40:31**

Early Diagnosis and Treatment Can Save Your Life

PART TWO

About You

Early Diagnosis and Treatment Can Save Your Life

What To Do
When You Don't Know
What To Do

Early Diagnosis and Treatment Can Save Your Life

Thinking about what you would do if you had cancer is very different from knowing what you need to do when you're diagnosed with it. No matter how much you've read, how much you've been told, or how much you think you know about it, you can never know too much about breast cancer. Situations will arise and you won't know what to do.

Make no mistake about it...fear is the enemy. Fear causes you to lose precious time; fear can cost you your life. It can manifest itself in a variety of ways including avoidance, extreme anxiety, procrastination, and denial. Don't let it dictate your future. When fear makes you weak, let knowledge make you strong. It is the best weapon against fear. One way to overcome the fear associated with this disease is to learn everything you possibly can about it.

This section is meant to educate, enlighten, and empower you. It contains virtually everything you need to know about breast cancer. It will provide you with enough information to make realistic and informed decisions regarding your health care. When you become better informed, you can actively participate in decisions that will have a positive and profound affect on your health and your life.

Early Diagnosis and Treatment Can Save Your Life

10
Dispelling The Myths; Understanding The Facts

Just as myths exist about almost everything else in life, breast cancer is no exception. Before you can begin to understand the impact of such a diagnosis, you must first separate fact from fiction. You have probably heard some of these myths.

I've certainly heard more than my share of "you know what they say" stories. In the first place, no one knows who "they" are and the mere fact that we believe in some of what "they" say is beyond comprehension. Nevertheless, we take a lot of these myths to heart. Sadly, some of these myths have caused so many women (and men) to lose their lives to this devastating disease.

Yes, even I've been guilty of basing a few of my decisions on things that I'd heard before getting proper information. At the time, these decisions seemed to be the right ones, but not necessarily the best ones. Before my diagnosis, I was totally ignorant when it came to breast cancer, and to some degree, my entire health. I was living one of the biggest myths of all: Breast cancer is a disease that isn't my concern. My diagnosis made me realize just how uninformed, unaware, and unprepared I was.

Early Diagnosis and Treatment Can Save Your Life

SOME SOBERING FACTS ABOUT BREAST CANCER

- **EVERY** woman is at risk for breast cancer.
- Breast cancer is the most common form of cancer in women in the United States.
- A new case of breast cancer is diagnosed every three minutes, and a woman will die from breast cancer every twelve minutes.
- Breast cancer is the second leading cause of cancer death for women between the ages of 35 and 54.
- Breast cancer incidence increases with age, rising sharply after age 40. About 80 percent of invasive breast cancers occur in women over age 50.
- Breast cancer is the leading cause of cancer death for African American women. While more white women are diagnosed with breast cancer, the mortality rate is higher among African American women.
- Women of low socioeconomic status are more likely to be diagnosed with late stage disease and die of it as a result.
- More than 80 percent of breast cancer cases occur in women who have no identifiable risk factors. Risk factors include:
    - Older than age 40, and especially older than 50.
    - Personal history of breast cancer (anyone who has had cancer in one breast).
    - Mother and/or sisters have had breast cancer, with the risk increasing if these relatives had cancer in both breasts, and it occurred before menopause.
    - Never having children or having first live birth after age 30.
    - Long menstrual history (periods started early and ended late in life).
    - Late menopause.
- The cause of breast cancer is unknown.
- There is nothing you can do to prevent getting breast cancer; however, you can minimize your risk.
- More than 80 percent of breast lumps are proven benign, but any breast lump must be evaluated by a physician.
- A cancer diagnosis is not a death sentence. You can live a happy, healthy and productive life after breast cancer. More than 2 million breast cancer survivors are alive in America today.

Early Diagnosis and Treatment Can Save Your Life

SOME COMMON MYTHS ABOUT BREAST CANCER

Myth: *You're too young to have breast cancer.*
Fact: Breast cancer knows no age barrier, although the disease is relatively uncommon in the 20s and more common in the 50s and 60s. According to the American Cancer Society, about 75 percent of women who get breast cancer are age fifty or older. But it's estimated that 9,000 American women, aged forty and younger, will be diagnosed with breast cancer. (I was diagnosed with breast cancer at age forty-two. The youngest person I met who had breast cancer was just twenty-three years old.) The good news is that, regardless of age, when breast cancer is found early, treatment is often extremely effective.

Myth: *Breast cancer is preventable.*
Fact: There is no certain way to prevent breast cancer, and the cause of the disease has not been determined. Early detection followed by prompt treatment offers the best chance to treat breast cancer successfully and to increase your chances of survival. It is true there are some things that you can do to minimize your risk; however, there are no known ways to prevent the disease from occurring.

Myth: *You don't have a family history of breast cancer, so you're not at risk.*
Fact: Hereditary breast cancer is the exception, and not the rule. It accounts for approximately 20 percent of cases. In the other 80 percent, there is no incidence of breast cancer in family history.

Myth: *Having a risk factor for breast cancer means you'll develop the disease.*
Fact: No risk factor, either alone or in combination with others, means you'll definitely get the disease. Some of these factors appear to increase your risk only slightly.

Myth: *Breast cancer is passed only from your mother, not your father.*
Fact: Experts now tell us that breast cancer genes can be inherited from your dad's side of the family as well. So it's important that you know medical histories on both sides of your family tree. (While I was the first to be diagnosed on my mother's side of the family; my daughter's aunt, her father's sister, had breast cancer as well.)

Early Diagnosis and Treatment Can Save Your Life

Myth: ***The statistic "one in eight" women will develop breast cancer means that if eight women are randomly selected, then one of the eight women is guaranteed to get breast cancer.***

Fact: The one-in-eight women statistic is not a per-year estimate. Rather it is calculated over a lifetime to age ninety-five. If researchers were to study a large group of girls born today and track them until they became 90 years old, then one out of every eight of those girls would develop breast cancer sometime in her lifetime.

Myth: ***Older women are less likely to get breast cancer than young women.***

Fact: As a woman's age increases, her risk of getting breast cancer also increases. In fact, age is one of the strongest risk factors for developing breast cancer. To help detect breast cancer early, women 40 years of age and older should get regular mammograms in addition to a yearly clinical breast examination and monthly breast self-exams. Women between the ages of 20 and 40 should also practice monthly breast self-exams and receive physician-performed clinical exams at least every three years.

A Woman's Chances of Breast Cancer Increases with Age	
By age 30	1 out of 2,212
By age 40	1 out of 235
By age 50	1 out of 54
By age 60	1 out of 23
By age 70	1 out of 14
By age 80	1 out of 10
Over 80	1 out of 8

Early Diagnosis and Treatment Can Save Your Life

Dispelling The Myths; Understanding The Facts

Myth: ***Only women get breast cancer.***
Fact: Not true. Although breast cancer in men is rare, men do get it. About 1,600 men are diagnosed each year and account for less than one percent of all breast cancers. Breast cancer kills about 25 percent of the men who develop it. While the statistics are low compared to the rate of breast cancer in women, it is important to know that men can get breast cancer also.

Myth: ***If I get breast cancer, I'm going to die.***
Fact: The number of women diagnosed with breast cancer has been rising substantially each year; however, the death rate has been steadily declining. Eighty percent of women diagnosed with breast cancer have no signs of metastases (no cancer has spread beyond the breast and nearby lymph nodes). Furthermore, 80 percent of these women live at least five years, and many live much longer. Even women with signs of cancer metastases can live a long time. Better treatments and early diagnosis through mammograms, clinical exams, and monthly breast self-exams are responsible for these improved outcomes.

Myth: ***In general, only white women get breast cancer.***
Fact: The truth is that although more white women are diagnosed with breast cancer, a greater percentage of African American women who have the disease will die of it. The rate of diagnosis is 13 percent higher among white women. But after five years, only 71 percent of African American women diagnosed with breast cancer are alive, compared to 86 percent of white women, according to the American Cancer Society. Most experts attribute the difference in survival rates to African American women's poorer access to health care. As a group, white, Hawaiian, and black women have the highest rates of the disease, according to the National Cancer Institute. The lowest rates occur among American Indian, Vietnamese, and Korean women.

Early Diagnosis and Treatment Can Save Your Life

Myth: **Eating high-fat foods causes breast cancer.**
Fact: A number of studies have found that women who live in countries where diets tend to be lower in fat have a lower risk of breast cancer. But the majority of studies focusing on women in the U.S. haven't found a solid link between dietary fat consumption and breast cancer risk. Why are these findings contradictory? It may be that women in other countries are at lower risk for other reasons: They exercise more, eat less, weigh less, smoke less, or have a different genetic profile or environmental interaction that makes them less susceptible. Postmenopausal obesity is a factor that does put you at risk for breast and other cancers, so it pays to maintain a healthy weight.

Myth: **Wearing a bra or using antiperspirants and deodorants increases your risk of breast cancer.**
Fact: It is absolutely not true that wearing a bra, especially underwire bras, traps toxins by limiting lymph and blood flow in your breasts, increasing risk. While sweat does contain water, urea, and salt, it does not contain toxins. There is also no proof for the claims that antiperspirants and deodorants cause cancer by keeping the body from sweating out the cancer-causing substances that build up in the breasts, or because they contain harmful chemicals that are absorbed through the skin. The sweat glands are not connected to the lymph nodes.

Myth: **I don't need a mammogram unless my health care professional says I do.**
Fact: Although most health care professionals remember to refer women for mammograms, you shouldn't wait for one to suggest it. The American Cancer Society recommends yearly mammograms for women age 40 and older. You should consult with your doctor if you detect a change in your breasts.

Myth: **I've had a normal mammogram so I don't need another.**
Fact: Once is not enough. Every woman age 40 or older should have an annual mammogram. Depending on how rapidly a tumor grows, mammography can detect it as much as two years before a manual exam can.

Early Diagnosis and Treatment Can Save Your Life

Dispelling The Myths; Understanding The Facts

Myth: *Mammograms can prevent breast cancer.*
Fact: While mammograms can detect breast cancer, they can't prevent it.

Myth: *If a mammogram does detect a problem, it's too late to do anything about it.*
Fact: Untrue. Mammograms can detect most breast cancers very early, giving you more treatment options and greater chances of survival.

Myth: *Mammograms aren't that helpful, and may be harmful.*
Fact: The best way to detect breast cancer at its earliest, most treatable stage, before it can be felt, is through safe, annual screening mammograms (breast x-rays) beginning at age 40. All U.S. mammography facilities must be inspected and government certified. Several studies have shown that regular mammography screenings can decrease a woman's chance of dying from breast cancer.

Myth: *Mammogram screening is unsafe.*
Fact: It is generally agreed that the risk from the radiation women are exposed to by annual, state-of-the-art mammography is negligible. Although there has been considerable controversy about the safety of mammography in the mid-1970s, it's quite different today. To be sure mammography is state-of-the art and to maintain stringent criteria of accuracy and quality with the extremely low level of radiation now being used, the American College of Radiology (ACR) began a voluntary accreditation program in 1987. The Mammography Quality Standards Act became effective in 1994. All mammography facilities must meet certain quality standards established by the Food and Drug Administration (FDA).

Myth: *If you have small breasts, you're much less likely to get breast cancer.*
Fact: Size doesn't matter. Any woman with breasts can get it. The amount of breast tissue a woman has does not affect her risk of developing breast cancer.

Early Diagnosis and Treatment Can Save Your Life

Myth: Breast cancer is contagious (spread by air, drinking from the cup of someone with the disease, etc.).
Fact: Cancer is not a communicable disease. Breast cancer is defined as an abnormal increase in breast cells, resulting in a malignant (cancerous) tumor of the breast tissue.

Myth: Breast-feeding can cause breast cancer.
Fact Breast-feeding does not cause breast cancer. In fact, some preliminary studies reveal that breast-feeding may decrease a woman's risk of developing breast cancer. However, this data has not been confirmed. Women who breast feed can still get breast cancer, but the risk is no more than that of women who do not breast feed.

Myth: An injury to the breast causes cancer.
Fact: Injury or trauma to the breast does not cause breast cancer. However, breasts may become bruised or develop a benign (non-cancerous) lump as a result of an injury.

Myth: Using an electric blanket can cause breast cancer.
Fact: The Nurse's Health Study of 8,497 women found no link between electric blankets and breast cancer.

Myth: Chemotherapy for breast cancer can be worse than the disease.
Fact: Chemotherapy and hormonal therapy (drugs to treat cancer) are increasingly recommended to improve survival. New, effective drugs that control chemotherapy's side effects help many women lead normal work and home lives during treatment.

Early Diagnosis and Treatment Can Save Your Life

11
Know Your Breasts

Getting to know your breasts is the first step in taking a role in their care and health. It is important to know what your breasts feel like, what they should look like, and to be aware of any abnormalities or changes in them. Understanding what changes occur in our breasts as we age is one of the simplest ways in which you can contribute to your self-care.

Early Diagnosis and Treatment Can Save Your Life

YOUR BREASTS

The size and shape of the breasts depend upon heredity, body weight, and supporting ligaments, and they do not necessarily match each other. If the fibrous tissue of the breast is high, the breasts will feel firm and retain their shape. When there is more fatty tissue, breasts are heavy or pendulous and feel softer.

What You See From The Outside
- The areola is the darker circle of skin surrounding each nipple.
- Hair sometimes grows out of the skin surrounding each areola.
- The nipple is the outlet for ducts carrying milk during breast-feeding.
- The inframammary crease, or bra line, is the thick fold beneath each breasts.

What You See From The Inside
- The breastbone runs down the center of your chest.
- The hard collarbone runs from each shoulder to your upper middle chest.
- Ribs are ridge like bones below your breast tissue.
- Firm muscles under your breast help you move your arms.
- Axillary lymph nodes feel soft and rubbery, and help defend your body against infection.
- Fatty tissue makes your breasts feel soft.
- Mammary glands produce milk and can feel lumpy.
- Ducts are tube-shaped structures that carry milk from your mammary glands to your nipples.
- Fibrous tissue supports your breasts, making them feel firm.

The breasts are milk-producing, tear-shaped glands. They are supported by and attached to the front of the chest wall on either side of the breast bone or sternum by ligaments. They rest on the major chest muscle, the pectoralis major. The breast has no muscle tissue, but muscles lie under each breast and cover the ribs. A layer of fat surrounds the glands and extends throughout the breast.

Each breast has 15 to 20 sections, called *lobes,* that are arranged like the petals of a daisy. Each lobe has many smaller *lobules*, which end in dozens of tiny *bulbs* that can produce milk. The lobes, lobules, and bulbs are all lined

Early Diagnosis and Treatment Can Save Your Life

Know Your Breasts *131*

by thin tubes called ***ducts***. These ducts lead to the nipple in the center of a dark area of skin called the areola. Fat fills the spaces between lobules and ducts.

Each breast also contains blood vessels and vessels that carry ***lymph***. The lymph vessels lead to small bean-shaped organs called ***lymph nodes***. Clusters of lymph nodes are found under the arm, above the collarbone, and in the chest, as well as in many other parts of the body.

Early Diagnosis and Treatment Can Save Your Life

Looking from the Outside In

Just as fingerprints are unique, so are each woman's breasts. That's why it's so important to get to know your own breasts—from the outside in—so you can tell what's normal for you. Learning about breast anatomy can help you more easily identify what you're seeing and feeling in your breasts when you do BSE. Knowing what changes to expect each month or as you grow older will make you more aware of any abnormal changes that may require medical attention.

What You See

The areola is the darker circle of skin surrounding each nipple.

Hair commonly grows out of the skin surrounding each areola.

The nipple is the outlet for ducts carrying milk during breastfeeding.

The inframammary crease, or bra line, is the thick fold beneath each breast.

Early Diagnosis and Treatment Can Save Your Life

Know Your Breasts 133

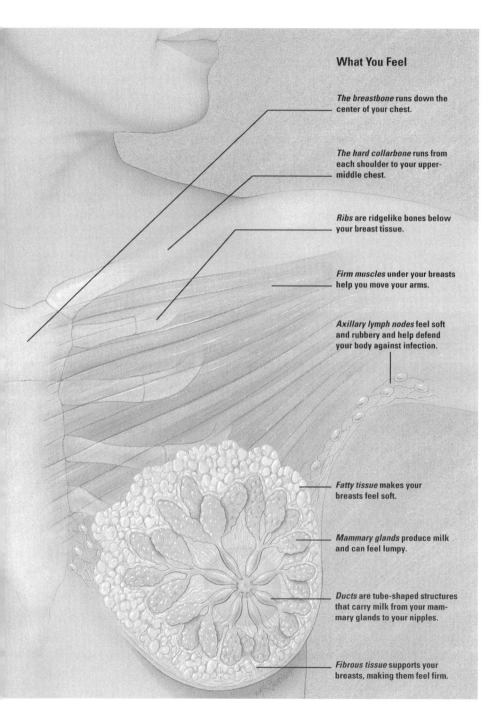

Early Diagnosis and Treatment Can Save Your Life

UNDERSTANDING NORMAL BREASTS CHANGES

Puberty
Normal changes in the breasts, including enlargement of the areola, begin when the breasts begin to grow. When the ovaries start to secrete estrogen, fat in the connective tissue begins to accumulate, causing the breasts to enlarge. The duct system also begins to grow. The maturing of the breasts begins with the formation of secretionary glands at the end of the milk ducts. The breasts and duct system continue to grow and mature, with the development of many glands and lobules. Growth is controlled by the female hormones estrogen and progesterone, which continue to produce normal changes in breast tissue throughout a woman's lifetime. The rate at which breasts grow varies greatly and is different for each young woman.

Menstrual Cycle
Each month, women experience fluctuations in hormones that make up the normal menstrual cycle. Estrogen, which is produced by the ovaries in the first half of the menstrual cycle, stimulates the growth of milk ducts in the breasts. The increasing level of estrogen leads to ovulation halfway though the cycle, and then the hormone progesterone takes over in the second half of the cycle, stimulating the formation of the milk glands. These hormones are believed to be responsible for the cyclical changes such as the swelling, pain, and tenderness that many women experience in their breasts just before menstruation.

During Pregnancy
Breast changes are one of the earliest signs of pregnancy—a result of the milk producing hormone, progesterone. Your mammary glands enlarge in preparation for milk production, making your breasts larger and firmer. Most pregnant women experience tenderness down the sides of the breasts and tingling or soreness of the nipples because of the growth of the milk duct system and the formation of the many more lobules. By the fourth or sixth month of pregnancy, the breasts are fully

Early Diagnosis and Treatment Can Save Your Life

capable of producing milk. Other changes, such as the prominence of the blood vessels in the breasts and the enlargement and darkening of the areola occur.

With Age
Over time, your breasts change in texture and appearance. Your ducts and mammary glands shrink after menopause and are replaced by fatty tissue, making your breasts feel less lumpy.

Menopause
Mammary glands decrease in size, fibrous breast tissue loses strength and elasticity and breasts become softer and sag with age. The skin of the breasts, normally smooth, may become wrinkled and the supporting ligaments slacken.

Weight Changes
Like other parts of the body that contain fatty tissue, your breasts may change in size or shape if you lose or gain weight.

BREAST CONDITIONS

Most breast conditions are benign, or non-cancerous, causing no serious harm to you. Even so, you can't know for sure until you've been evaluated by your health care professional. All women are at some risk for breast cancer, especially as they become older. If you experience any breast changes, be sure to have an evaluation.

Benign Breasts Lumps
Most breast lumps are benign (with harmless causes). Benign breast lumps usually have smooth edges, can be moved slightly when you push against them, and come in all shapes, textures, and sizes. They are often found in both breasts. There are several causes for benign lumps, including normal changes in breast tissue, breast infection or injury and medicines that may cause lumps or breast pain. If a lump is benign it

Early Diagnosis and Treatment Can Save Your Life

may not need treatment unless it causes symptoms that bother you. Common causes for benign breast lumps include fibrocystic changes, cysts, and glandular tissue (fibroadenoma). These lumps usually feel smooth, firm, and rubbery, and are painless and movable.

Fibrocystic Condition
For many women, fluctuations in hormones during normal monthly menstrual cycles can create changes in the breasts that are referred to as fibrocystic breast changes. Women with fibrocystic breasts usually experience lumps in both breasts that increase in size and tenderness just prior to menstrual bleeding. The cysts rapidly enlarge in response to hormones released near menstruation. They occasionally have nipple discharge as well. The lumps may be hard or rubbery and may be felt as a single (large or small) breast lump. Fibrocystic changes can also cause thickening of the breast tissue. These symptoms are typically somewhat relieved at the end of menstruation.

Cysts
A cyst is a fluid-filled sac that can feel like a lump. Cysts may form due to hormonal changes and usually occur in both breasts. You may have one or more. Cystic lumps range in size and often feel smooth, somewhat like a small water balloon. Cysts can become larger and more painful every month right before your period. They often feel less painful and get smaller after your period. The fluid inside a cyst may be aspirated (drained).

Fibroadenoma
Fibroadenomas are the most common benign tumors found in the female breasts. A fibroadenoma is a knot of fibrous and mammary gland tissue. They are solid, round, rubbery lumps that move freely in the breast when pushed upon and are usually painless. Fibroadenomas are the result of excess formation of lobules (milk-producing glands) and surrounding breast tissue. They occur most often between the ages of 20 and 30 and are more common in African-American women. A

Early Diagnosis and Treatment Can Save Your Life

fibroadenoma can feel sore or tender, becoming more painful just before each period. Sometimes, though, it causes no pain. Your health care provider may suggest that a fibroadenoma be removed.

Fat Necrosis
Painless, round, and firm lumps formed by damaged and disintegrating fatty tissues. This condition typically occurs in obese women with very large breasts. It often develops in response to a bruise or blow to the breasts. Sometimes the skin around the lumps looks red or bruised. Fat necrosis can easily be mistaken for cancer, so such lumps are removed in a surgical biopsy.

Sclerosing Adenois
A benign condition involving the excessive growth of tissues in the breast's lobules. It frequently causes breast pain. Usually the changes are microscopic, but adenosis can produce lumps, and it can show up on mammography, often as calcifications. Short of biopsy, adenosis can be difficult to distinguish from cancer. The usual approach is surgical biopsy, which furnishes both diagnosis and treatment.

Intraductal Papillomas
Small wart-like growths that grow in the lining of the mammary ducts, near the nipple. Any slight bump or bruise in the area of the nipple can cause the papilloma to bleed. Single (solitary) intraductal papillomas usually affect women nearing menopause. If the discharge becomes bothersome, the diseased duct can be removed surgically without damaging the appearance of the breast. Multiple intraductal papillomas are more common in younger women. They often occur in both breasts and are more likely to be associated with a lump than with nipple discharge. Multiple intraductal papillomas, or any papillomas associated with a lump, need to be removed.

Calcifications
Calcifications are deposits of calcium in one or both breasts. These deposits can be seen only with a mammogram. On a mammogram, cal-

Early Diagnosis and Treatment Can Save Your Life

cifications look like tiny white specks. Most of the time, they are benign. Certain patterns of calcifications, though, can indicate breast cancer. Your health care provider may want to do further testing if calcifications are found.

Nipple Discharge
Many women can squeeze a tiny amount of a clear, greenish, or milky discharge from both nipples, a perfectly normal condition, and is more common among women who have given birth. A pinkish discharge can be caused by a benign growth (intraductal papilloma) in a duct near the nipple. If a discharge is bloody or spontaneous (happening without squeezing your nipples), be sure to have it checked by your health care provider.

Breast Infection
One of the most common types of breast infection is mastitis (sometimes called "postpartum mastitis"). This infection is most often seen in women who are breast-feeding. A duct may become blocked, allowing milk to pool, causing inflammation and setting the stage for infection by bacteria. The breast appears red and feels warm, tender, and lumpy. In its earlier stages, mastitis can be cured by antibiotics. If a pus containing abscess forms, it will need to be drained or surgically removed.

Mammary Duct Ectasia (Ek-ta'ze-a)
A disease of women nearing menopause. Ducts beneath the nipple become inflamed and can become clogged. Mammary duct ectasia can become painful, and it can produce a thick and sticky discharge that is gray to green in color. Treatment consists of warm compresses, antibiotics, and, if necessary, surgery to remove the duct.

Costochondritis (Kos'to-kon-dri'tis)
Costochondritis is swelling and inflammation in the ribs underneath the breast. The pain may feel worse when you take a deep breath. The cause is unknown, but it may be more common in women with large breasts

Early Diagnosis and Treatment Can Save Your Life

Costochondritis heals over time. Ibuprofen or aspirin often helps relieve the pain.

Note: Don't use this information to self-diagnose. Should you have or think you have one or more of these conditions, have your physician evaluate it.

Early Diagnosis and Treatment Can Save Your Life

12

Screening And Warning Signs

Breast cancer is not something a woman "gets" or "catches," like a case of the mumps. Breast cancer develops over time, beginning with one tiny abnormal cell. Sometimes the development takes a long time. At other times, the type of cancer can be very aggressive and the tumors develop quickly. Any change in the shape, texture (raised, thickened skin for example), or color of the skin should be examined by a physician. The earlier breast cancer is found, the better the chances for successful treatment and survival.

Understanding the normal anatomy of your breasts will help you to become familiar with the normal feel of them and to gain confidence in your ability to do a breast self-exam (BSE) correctly. By performing monthly BSE you will be able to distinguish between suspicious new lumps and ordinary breast tissue that sometimes feels lumpy. BSE is relatively simple and requires only a little bit of your time once a month. This procedure should also become second nature to you. Whether you do it in the shower, lying on the bed, on the floor, in a circular, line, or wedge pattern...JUST DO IT AND LEARN HOW TO DO IT CORRECTLY. (For those of you who are a tad more uninhibited than others, get your significant other involved in checking your breasts; it can be a lot of fun!) Performing a breast exam is far less time-consuming than visiting the doctor, hospitals, your oncologist, and other breast care specialists.

A mammogram and a professional clinical exam are the two other elements that complete the process for healthy breasts. Depending on your age, family history, and other factors, you should start having these two procedures done on a regular basis also. When to have a mammogram and/or professional clinical exam is discussed in the summary of the American Cancer Society Guidelines that follow.

Early Diagnosis and Treatment Can Save Your Life

Screening and Warning Signs

BREAST SELF-EXAMINATION (BSE)

Unfortunately, many women avoid breast self-exams altogether. Fear, embarrassment, inexperience, or simply not remembering to do it are a few of the reasons. The arguments for doing BSE are stronger. By performing BSE you're simply giving yourself a head start against potential trouble. You can know the "landscape" of your breast better than anyone else. And with monthly practice, you can become skilled at looking and feeling for changes in your breasts.

The American Cancer Society recommends that all women over the age of 20 examine their breasts once a month. BSE is recommended because noticeable breast cancer symptoms can develop between clinical breast exams and mammography.

It is important for you to be familiar with your breasts so that you can learn the texture of your normal tissue and be able to recognize any changes. By doing self examination each month, you can improve your skill at feeling different structures in your breast tissue. Breast self-examination is an important part of breast cancer screening since most cancers are still detected by women themselves. This is true despite the availability of mammography and clinical breast exams. A lump first found by mammography is usually smaller than the one first found by BSE. However, lumps found by women who do breast self-exams regularly are usually smaller than those found by chance. NOTE: The following is a dramatization.

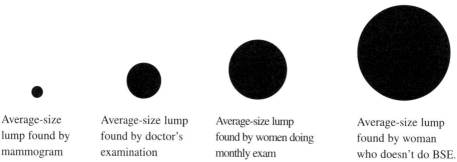

| Average-size lump found by mammogram | Average-size lump found by doctor's examination | Average-size lump found by women doing monthly exam | Average-size lump found by woman who doesn't do BSE. |

Early Diagnosis and Treatment Can Save Your Life

BSE is a simple skill that costs no money, takes little time, and may save your life. If you perform BSE carefully at the same time each month, you can become familiar with the landscape of your breasts. Knowing how your breasts usually feel can help you notice any unusual changes, such as a thickening or lump, before it goes beyond the early stages. The American Cancer Society recommends that premenopausal women examine their breasts when they are least tender, usually one week after menstruation starts. Postmenopausal women should do so the first day of every month. If you notice any unusual changes, make an appointment to see your health care professional. Breast-feeding mothers should examine their breasts when all milk has been expressed. Nine out of ten women will not develop breast cancer and most breast changes are not cancerous; however, if you discover a lump or detect any changes, you should seek medical attention immediately.

<u>Technique</u>

- Use the pads of the three middle fingers and hold hand in bowed position.
- Examine entire area using vertical strip pattern.
- Examine area from underarm to lower bra line, across to breast bone, up to collar bone, and back to armpit.

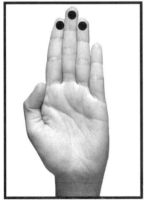 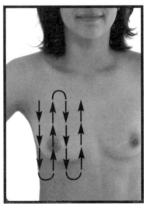 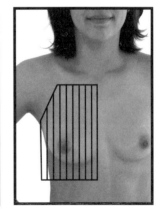

Early Diagnosis and Treatment Can Save Your Life

Screening and Warning Signs   *143*

Simple 1-2-3 of Breast Exam

1. At the Mirror

Stand in front of your mirror. First, view your breasts with you hands relaxed at your sides, then with hands clasped behind your head. Look for lumps, dimpling, rash, or puckering of the skin or nipple. Repeat with hands on your hips, flexing your chest muscles. Then, gently squeeze each nipple between your thumb and forefingerm, checking for a sticky or obviously bloody discharge. A drop or two of clear milky fluid is normal.

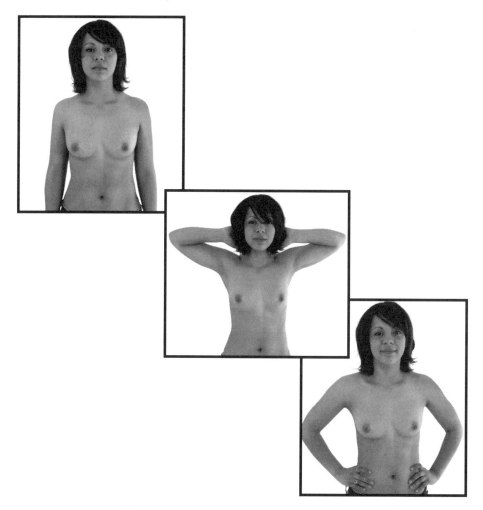

Early Diagnosis and Treatment Can Save Your Life

144   *Breastlessness*

2. **In The Shower**

Wet, soapy skin makes this step easier. Raise your left arm overhead and mentally divide your entire breast into a series of vertical or horizontal strips. Hold the middle fingers of your right hand flat against your left breast. Starting at the center of your armpit, press straight down and move your fingers in small circular motions. Continue up and down the strips as though mowing the lawn. Use light, medium, and deep pressure in each spot to probe the entire depth of breast tissue.

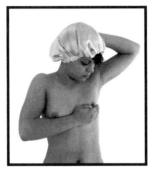

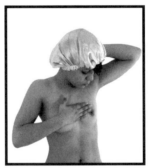

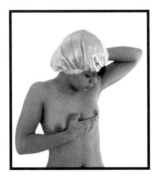

Early Diagnosis and Treatment Can Save Your Life

Screening and Warning Signs 145

Lying Down

Put a pillow under your left shoulder to help flatten the breast evenly over your chest. This allows you to examine the breast tissue by pressing against the firm chest wall. With your left arm above your head, begin at the armpit and make three small circles. Each about the size of a dime. Use light, medium, and firm pressure. Examine area from underarm to lower bra line, across to breastbone, up to collarbone and back to arm pit, using a vertical strip pattern.

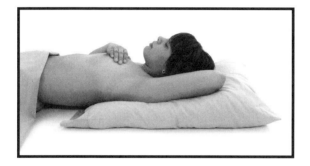

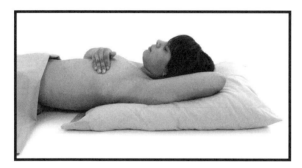

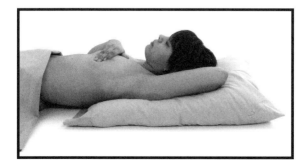

Early Diagnosis and Treatment Can Save Your Life

Plan of Action

Every woman should have a personal breast health plan of action:

Discuss the American Cancer Society's breast cancer detection guidelines with your health professional.

Schedule your clinical breast exam and mammogram as appropriate for your age.

Perform monthly breast self examinations. Ask your health professional for feedback on your BSE skills.

Report any breast changes to your health professional.

Early Diagnosis and Treatment Can Save Your Life

MAMMOGRAM

Mammogram is a special kind of x-ray. It is different from a chest x-ray or x-rays of other parts of the body. Mammography involves two x-rays of each breasts, one taken from the side and one from the top.

Each breast is compressed with a plastic shield, sponge, or balloon. Then two or three x-rays are taken of each breast.

A radiologist examines the x-rays and reports to your doctor. The mammogram should not hurt; however, there is slight discomfort, particularly when x-raying small breasts. A mammogram can detect breast cancer even before a lump is large enough for you or your health care provider to feel.

Improved detection methods have led to earlier detection of breast cancer when the tumor is small. At this early stage breast cancer is more easily and successfully treated. Doctors and their patients now can plan individualized treatment using surgery and, if appropriate, radiation therapy, chemotherapy, and hormones.

There is no universal agreement on screening policy for younger women, with regard to either the age at which to begin or the frequency of subsequent mammograms. Several, but not all, national and professional organizations in the United States recommend that all women over the age of forty should be screened at regular intervals. Others recommend that routine mammography begin at age fifty. The American Cancer Society recommends that women age 40 and over should have a screening mammogram every year and should continue to do so for as long as they are in good health. If your mother or sister has had breast cancer, talk to your health care provider about when you should start having mammograms.

Early Diagnosis and Treatment Can Save Your Life

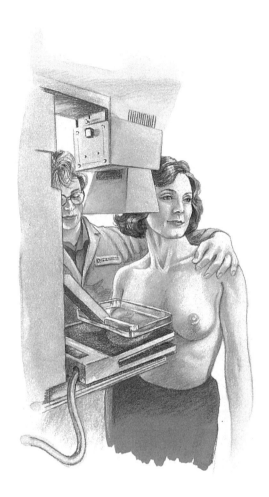

Important Note: *A negative mammogram does not exclude the possibility of breast disease. You should never ignore a breast lump or any other changes in your breasts, even if the mammogram is normal. If you should find a lump or other change, talk to your health care provider about it as soon as possible.*

Early Diagnosis and Treatment Can Save Your Life

Where to Get A Low Cost Or Free Mammogram

If you do not have health insurance, you have a number of other options:

- Call your local chapter of the American Cancer Society or the national toll-free number, 800-ACS-2345. The ACS will be able to tell you about any low-cost or free mammography programs that offer screening to women unable to pay for it themselves.

- Call your State Department of Health. Every state now has a **Breast and Cervical Early Detection Program** funded by the U.S. Centers for Disease Control and Prevention, planned or in operation. This program offers screening to qualifying women unable to pay for it themselves.

- Call the YWCA's ENCORE PLUS Program for access to low-cost or free mammograms. To find which YWCA facilities offer this service and if you are eligible, call 1 (800) 872-9622, your local YWCA.

- Call the National Cancer Institute at 800-4-CANCER for the names of FDA-certified, accredited mammography facilities in your area. If you explain your financial situation, some mammography facilities are willing to work out a lower fee or payment schedule that will make the test more affordable. Ask the facility if they are willing to discuss these options with you.

- Check with your local health departments. They can provide you with the names of clinics who offer mammograms free or for a reduced rate depending on financial ability to pay.

- October of each year is *National Breast Cancer Awareness Month*, and many mammography facilities offer special fees and extended hours during this month.

- Get a list of the names of support groups in your area. These groups contain a wealth of information on screening, testing, and other issues related to women's health.

Early Diagnosis and Treatment Can Save Your Life

Other Techniques for Detecting Breast Cancer

Blood tests. Some blood tests are needed to plan surgery, to screen for evidence of cancer spread, and to plant treatment after surgery. These blood tests include: **Complete blood count (CBC).** This determines whether the blood has the correct type and number of blood cells. Abnormal test results could reveal other health problems including anemia, and could suggest the cancer has spread to the bone marrow. **Blood chemical and enzyme tests.** These tests are done in patients with invasive breast cancer and may show the cancer has spread to the bone or liver. If these test results are higher than normal, your doctor will order imaging tests such as bone scans or CT scans.

Bone scan. This test helps show if cancer has spread to the bones. A radioactive substance is injected and collects in diseased bone cells throughout the body. These areas know as "hot spots." Arthritis, infection, or other bone diseases can also cause hot spots. Bone scans can find metastases much sooner than normal x-rays. Discuss this procedure with your physician as a regular screening tool.

Chest x-ray. All women with breast cancer should have a chest x-ray before surgery to make sure that the cancer has not spread to the lungs.

Computer Tomography, or CT scanning, uses a computer to organize the information from multiple x-ray views and construct a cross sectional image of the body. CT is sometimes helpful in locating breast lesions that are difficult to pinpoint with mammography or ultrasound—for instance, a tumor that is so close to the chest wall that it shows up in only one mammographic view.

Recently, it has become possible to identify ***Genetic Changes*** that predispose women to breast cancer. This type of molecular diagnostic test is made possible because scientists have precisely located the BRCA1 and BRCA2 genes, which normally work to control cell growth in breast tissue. When certain genetic changes called mutations occur in

Early Diagnosis and Treatment Can Save Your Life

these genes, a person may be more susceptible to developing breast cancer. Several newer techniques for imaging the breast are being used. These include:

Magnetic Resonance Imaging, or ***MRI***, which relies on magnetic fields and radio waves to produce a likeness of body tissues. ***Laser beam scanning*** shines a powerful laser beam through the breast while a special camera on the far side of the breast records the image.

Researchers are also striving to make mammography more sensitive and more accurate. ***Digital mammography*** is a technique for recording x-ray images in computer code, allowing the information to be manipulated in ways that enhance subtle, but potentially significant, variations. ***Computer-Aided Diagnosis,*** or ***CAD***, uses special computer programs to scan mammographic images and alert radiologists to areas that look suspicious.

Position Emission Tomography (PET). PET scans use a form of sugar (glucose) that contains a radioactive atom. A small amount of the radioactive materials is injected into your arm. Then you are put into the PET machine where a special camera can detect the radioactivity. Because of their high rate of metabolism, cancer cells of the body absorb large amounts of the radioactive sugar. PET scans can be used instead of several different x-rays because it scans your whole body.

Tumor tests (estrogen receptor, progesterone receptor, and HER-2/neu). Testing the tumor itself for certain substances helps determine the chances the cancer will spread, and helps the doctor determine the best treatment. Testing for hormone receptors helps determine the best treatment. Two hormones in women – estrogen and progesterone – may stimulate the growth of normal breast cells. Cancer cells respond to these hormones through the estrogen receptors (ER) and progesterone receptors (PR). ER and PR are the cell's "welcome mat" for these hormones circulating in the blood. If a cancer does not have these receptors, it is referred to as estrogen-receptor negative and/or progesterone-

***Early Diagnosis and Treatment Can Save Your Life**

receptor negative. If the cancer has these receptors, it is referred to as estrogen-receptor positive or just hormone-receptor positive (ER-positive, PR-positive).

Women with invasive breast cancer should also be tested for another receptor that helps cells grow. This is called HER-2-neu. Breast cancer cells with too much HER-2/neu tend to grow faster and may respond better to combinations of chemotherapy drugs in the anthracycline class (such as doxorubicin or epirubicin) and a drug that directly attacks HER-2/neu, an antibody called trastuzumab (Herceptin). Trastuzumab is not used unless it is known that the cancer has spread.

Ultrasound works by sending high-frequency sounds waves into the breast. The pattern of echoes from these sound waves is converted into an image (***sonogram***) of the breast's interior. Ultrasound, which is painless and harmless, is especially good in distinguishing between tumors that are solid and cysts, which are filled with fluid. Sonograms of the breast can also be helpful in evaluating some lumps that can be felt but are hard to see on a mammogram, especially in the dense breasts of young women. Unlike mammography, ultrasound cannot detect the microcalcifications that sometimes indicate cancer, nor does it pick up small tumors.

CLINICAL BREAST EXAM

Someone who is technically trained, such as your gynecologist or breast health specialist, should perform your professional breast exam. Backed by experience and knowledge, your health care professional may be more likely to notice a subtle change and know the appropriate tests and follow up care needed if an abnormality is found. You'll usually have a professional breast exam during the course of your regular checkup. Be sure to follow the ACS guidelines for regular exams.

During regular health checkups, you should have a professional breast examination. The health care provider should inspect your breasts look-

Early Diagnosis and Treatment Can Save Your Life

ing for changes in shape or unusual contour, spontaneous nipple discharge, skin dimpling, or other changes. After the visual exam, the area of the breasts, chest, and armpits should be palpated thoroughly to check for lumps or thickening.

At this time, you should observe how the health care provider carries out the exam, especially the amount of pressure applied. It is a good opportunity for you to ask for a description of what the health care provider feels, whether any changes are noted from the last exam, and other questions related to the current exam. You should also talk to your health care provider about your own risk for breast cancer and how often you should have a clinical breast examination.

The American Cancer Society recommends:

IF YOU ARE BETWEEN 20 AND 40 YEARS OLD
- Examine your breasts monthly.
- Get a clinical breast exam at least every three years.

IF YOU ARE BETWEEN 40 AND 49 YEARS OLD
- Examine your breasts monthly.
- Have a clinical breast exam every year.
- Have a mammogram every one to two years, starting at age 40.

IF YOU ARE 50 OR OLDER
- Examine your breasts monthly.
- Have a clinical breast exam every year.
- Have a mammogram every year.

Good breast care involves a combination of three important steps: a monthly breast self-examination, an annual examination by a health care professional and periodic mammograms.

Early Diagnosis and Treatment Can Save Your Life

BREAST CANCER WARNING SIGNS

When cancer is present, it is important that you be seen by a physician as soon as possible. Become familiar with early signs of cancer. Not only are there different types of breast cancer, but there are various stages in which cancer is diagnosed. There are aggressive cancers; there are rare cancers. Many of us are familiar with the lump as a possible sign of cancer, but there are other signs as well.

Early detection of breast cancer could save your life. Don't procrastinate, don't ignore it, and don't fear it. If you discover a lump or any one of the other cancer warning signs, see a physician as soon as possible.

Early Diagnosis and Treatment Can Save Your Life

Screening And Warning Signs   *155*

Consult your healthcare professional if you find any of the following during your self-exam or at any other time:

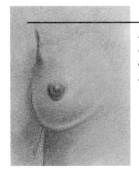

Distinct single lumps that are either hard or soft.

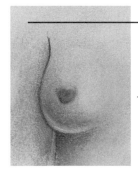

Changes in breast shape such as dimpling (depression), bulges, or flattening.

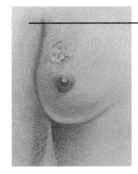

Changes in skin texture or color, including redness, "orange peel" (pebbly) skin, thickening, roughness, or puckering.

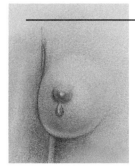

Bloody or cloudy nipple discharge.

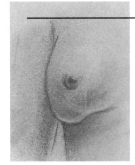

Changes in nipple location or shape.

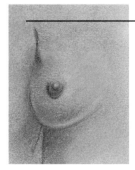

Breast sores that don't heal.

Early Diagnosis and Treatment Can Save Your Life

WHAT IS BREAST CANCER?

Breast cancer is an abnormal growth of the cells that line the ducts and the lobules. Breast cancer is classified by whether the cancer started in the ducts or the lobules, whether the cells have "invaded" (grown or spread) through the duct or lobule, and the way the cancer cells look under a microscope.

TYPES OF BREAST CANCER

Carcinoma In Situ
In situ means that the cancer is still in the ducts or lobules where it started and has not spread into surrounding fatty tissues in the breast or to other organs in the body. There are two types of breast carcinoma in situ:

Lobular Carcinoma In Situ (LCIS) Also called lobular neoplasia. It begins in the lobules, but does not grow through the lobule walls. Most breast cancer specialists think that LCIS, itself, does not usually become an invasive cancer, but women with this condition do run a higher risk of developing an invasive cancer in either breast.

Ductal Carcinoma In Situ (DCIS) The most common type of noninvasive breast cancer. Cancer cells inside the ducts do not spread through the walls of the ducts into the fatty tissue of the breast. These are treated with surgery and sometimes radiation, which are usually curative. Having untreated DCIS greatly increases the risk of invasive breast cancer.

Infiltrating (or Invasive Ductal Carcinoma)
The cancer starts in a milk passage, or duct, or the breast, but then the cancer cells break through the wall of the duct and spread into the breast's fatty tissue. They can then invade lymphatic channels or blood vessels of the breast and spread to other parts of the body. About 80% of all breast cancers are infiltrating or invasive ductal carcinoma.

Early Diagnosis and Treatment Can Save Your Life

Infiltrating (or Invasive Lobular Carcinoma)
This type of cancer starts in the milk-producing glands. Like infiltrating ductal breast cancer, this cancer can spread beyond the breast to other parts of the body. About 10% to 15% of invasive breast cancers are invasive lobular carcinomas.

Medullar Carcinoma
This special type of infiltrating ductal cancer has a relatively well-defined, distinct boundary between tumor tissue and normal breast tissue. It also has a number of other special features, including the large size of the cancer cells and the presence of immune system cells at the edges of the tumor. It accounts for about 5% of all breast cancers.

Colloid Carcinoma
This rare type of invasive ductal breast cancer, also called mucinous carcinoma, is formed by mucus-producing cancer cells. Colloid carcinoma has a slightly better prognosis and a slightly lower chance of metastasis than invasive lobular or invasive ductal cancers of the same size.

Tubular Carcinoma
Tubular carcinoma is a special type of infiltrating ductal breast carcinoma. About 2% of all breast cancers are tubular carcinomas. Women with this type of breast cancer have a better outlook because the cancer is less likely to spread outside the breast than invasive lobular or invasive ductal cancers of the same size.

Inflammatory Breast Cancer
This uncommon type of invasive breast cancer accounts for about 1-3% of all breast cancers. The skin of the affected breast is red, feels warm, and has the appearance of an orange peel. Doctors now know that these changes are not caused by inflammation, but by cancer cells blocking lymph vessels in the skin.

Inflammatory breast cancer has a higher chance of spreading and a worse prognosis than typical invasive ductal or lobular cancers. Inflammatory breast cancer is always staged as stage IIIB unless it has already spread to other organs at the time of diagnosis, which would then make it stage IV.

Early Diagnosis and Treatment Can Save Your Life

BREAST CANCER STAGES

Staging a cancer is the process of finding out how far the cancer has progressed when it is diagnosed. Doctors determine the stage of a cancer by gathering information from examinations and tests on the tumor, lymph nodes, and distant organs. A breast cancer's stage is one of the most important factors in predicting prognosis (outlook) or the chance of cancer coming back or spreading to other organs. Therefore, a cancer's stage is important in choosing the best treatment.

Each woman's outlook with breast cancer differs, depending on the cancer's stage and other factors such as hormone receptors, her general state of health, and her treatment.

Early Diagnosis and Treatment Can Save Your Life

Specific Stages of Breast Cancer

Stage 0	Very early breast cancer. This type of cancer has notspread within or outside the breast. It is sometimes called DCIS, LCIS, or breast cancer in situ or non invasive cancer.
Stage I	The cancer is no larger than about 1 inch, and has not spread outside the breast.
Stage II	The doctor may find any of the following: The cancer is no larger than 1 inch, but has spread to the lymph nodes under the arm. The cancer is between 1 inch and 2 inches; it may or may not have spread to the lymph nodes under the arm. The cancer is larger than 2 inches, but has not spread to the lymph nodes under the arm.
Stage III	This stage is divided into stages IIIA and IIIB:
Stage IIIA	The doctor may find either of the following: The cancer is smaller than 2 inches and has spread to the lymph nodes under the arm. The cancer also is spreading further to other lymph nodes. The cancer is larger than 2 inches and has spread to the lymph nodes under the arm.
Stage IIIB	The doctor may find either of the following: The cancer has spread to tissues near the breast (skin, chest wall, including the ribs and the muscles in the chest). The cancer has spread to lymph nodes inside the chest wall along the breast bone.
Stage IV	The cancer has spread to other parts of the body, most often the bones, lungs, liver or brain. Or, the tumor has spread locally to the skin and lymph nodes inside the neck, near the collarbone.
Inflammatory Breast Cancer	Inflammatory breast cancer is rare, but is a very aggressive type of cancer. The breast may look red and feel warm. You may see ridges, welts, or hives on your breast; or the skin may look wrinkled. It is sometimes misdiagnosed as a simple infection.

Early Diagnosis and Treatment Can Save Your Life

Recurrent Breast Cancer   Recurrent disease means that the cancer has come back after is has been treated. It may come back in the breast, in the soft cancer tissues of the chest (the chest wall), or in another part of the body.

HOW TO FIND A BREAST SPECIALIST

Women should select a board-certified surgical breast specialist or surgical oncologist to perform a surgical biopsy of a suspicious mass, or for further surgery once breast cancer has been confirmed by biopsy. A confirmed diagnosis of breast cancer should not be considered a medical emergency that must be treated immediately, although prompt surgical treatment (within a few weeks from diagnosis) is recommended. A patient should not hesitate to spend time locating a specialist, and consulting with other physicians for a second opinion. Take the time you need to make a sound decision.

To find a breast specialist:

- Ask your family doctor or gynecologist for a referral. Your doctor can also contact the American Society of Clinical Oncology to be referred to local surgical oncologists who are ASCO members. The American Board of Medical Specialists at 866-275-2267 can verify a physician's board certification by specialty and year, and will refer callers to local board-certified doctors.

- Call the National Cancer Institute's Cancer Information Service at 800-4CANCER for the names of NCI affiliated Clinical or Comprehensive Cancer Centers in your state, or members of the NCI's CCOI program. If none of these centers is conveniently located, call the department of surgery at the nearest one and ask for a local referral.

- Ask-A-Nurse is a free service providing 24-hour health care information and referrals from registered nurses in select locations around the country. Call 800-535-1111 to find out if there is an office in your area.

Early Diagnosis and Treatment Can Save Your Life

- Call the American Society of Plastic Surgeons referral service at 888-475-2784 and ask for a list of board certified plastic surgeons.

- If you know someone who has had breast cancer, ask her if she was pleased with her doctor. If so, ask her if the physician is accepting new patients and use her as a referral.

WHAT TO EXPECT WHEN YOU FIND A LUMP

If you discover a lump in one breast, examine the other breast. If both breasts feel the same, the lumpiness is probably normal. You should, however, mention it to your doctor at your next visit.

But if the lump is something new or unusual and does not go away after your menstrual period, it is time to call your doctor. The same is true if you discover a discharge from the nipple or skin changes such as dimpling or puckers. You should not let fear delay you. It's natural to be concerned if you find a lump in your breast. It's important to remember that 80 percent of all breast lumps are benign, which means no cancer is present. The sooner any problem is diagnosed, the sooner you can have it treated.

Clinical Evaluation

No matter how your breast lump is discovered, the doctor will want to begin your medical history. Your doctor will probably ask questions such as what symptoms do you have and how long have you had them? What is your age, menstrual status, general health? Are you pregnant? Are you taking any medications? How many children do you have? Do you have any relatives with benign breast conditions or breast cancer? Have you previously been diagnosed with benign breast changes?

The doctor will then carefully examine your breasts and will probably schedule you for diagnostic mammogram. If you have a symptom suggestive of breast cancer, you should not hesitate to have a mammogram if your doctor recommends it.

Early Diagnosis and Treatment Can Save Your Life

Aspirating a Cyst

When a cyst is suspected, some doctors proceed directly with *aspiration*. This procedure, which uses a very thin needle and a syringe, takes only a few minutes and can be done in the doctor's office. The procedure is not usually very uncomfortable, since most of the nerves in the breast are in the skin.

Holding the lump steady, the doctor inserts the needle and attempts to draw out any fluid. If the lump is indeed a cyst, removing the fluid will cause the cyst to collapse and the lump to disappear. Unless the cyst reappears in the next week or two, no other treatment is needed. If the cyst reappears at a later date, it can simply be drained again.

If the lump turns out to be solid, it may be possible to use the needle to withdraw a clump of cells, which can then be sent to a laboratory for further testing. (Cysts are so rarely associated with cancer that the fluid removed from a cyst is not usually tested unless it is bloody, or the woman is older than 55 years of age.)

Biopsy

The only definitive way to learn whether a breast lump or mammographic abnormality is cancerous is by having a *biopsy,* a procedure in which tissue is removed by a surgeon or other specialist and examined under a microscope by a pathologist. The pathologist is a physician who specializes in identifying tissue changes that are characteristic of disease, including cancer.

Tissue samples for a biopsy can be obtained either by surgery or needle. The doctor's choice of biopsy technique depends on such things as the nature and location of the lump as well as the woman's general health.

Surgical biopsies can be either excisional or incisional.

- An *excisional biopsy* removes the lump or the suspicious area in its entirety. Excision is currently the standard procedure for biopsying lumps that are smaller than an inch or so in diameter. In effect it is

Early Diagnosis and Treatment Can Save Your Life

similar to a "lumpectomy," surgery to remove the lump and a margin of surrounding tissue. Lumpectomy is usually used in combination with radiotherapy as the basic treatment for early breast cancer.

An excisional biopsy is typically performed in the outpatient department of a hospital. A local anesthetic is injected into the woman's breast. Sometimes, she is given a tranquilizer before the procedure. The surgeon makes an incision along the contour of the breast and removes the lump along with a small margin of normal tissue. Because no skin is removed, the biopsy scar is usually small. The procedure typically takes less than an hour. After spending an hour or two in the recovery room, the woman goes home the same day.

- An *incisional biopsy* removes only a portion of the tumor (by slicing into or incising it) for the pathologist to examine. Incisional biopsies are generally reserved for tumors that are larger. They too are usually performed under local anesthesia, with the woman going home the same day.

Whether or not a surgical biopsy will change the shape of your breast depends partly on the size of the lump and where it is located in the breast as well as how much of a "margin" of healthy tissue the surgeon decides to remove. You should talk with your doctor beforehand so you understand just how extensive the surgery will be and what the cosmetic result will be.

- *Needle biopsies* can be performed with either a very fine needle or a cutting needle large enough to remove a small nugget of tissue.

- *Fine needle aspiration*, as noted above, uses a fine-gauge needle and syringe, either to remove fluid from a cyst or cluster of cells from a solid mass. Accurate fine-needle aspiration biopsy of a solid mass takes great skill, gained through experience with numerous cases.

- *Core needle biopsy* uses a somewhat larger needle with a special cutting edge. The needle is inserted, under local anesthesia, through a small incision in the skin, and a small core of tissue is removed. This technique may not work well for lumps that are very hard or very small. Core needle biopsy may cause some bruising, but rarely leaves an

Early Diagnosis and Treatment Can Save Your Life

external scar, and the procedure is over in a matter of minutes.

At some institutions with extensive experience, aspiration biopsy is considered as reliable as surgical biopsy, trusted to confirm the malignancy of a clinically suspicious mass or, alternatively, to support a benign diagnosis for a breast lump that appears non-cancerous. Should the needle biopsy results be uncertain, the diagnosis is pursued with a surgical biopsy. At some institutions, doctors prefer to verify all aspiration biopsy results with a surgical biopsy before proceeding with treatment.

- *Localization biopsy* (also known as needle localization) is a procedure that uses mammography to locate the biopsy breast abnormalities that can be seen on a mammogram but cannot be felt (nonpalpable abnormalities). Localization can be used in conjunction with surgical biopsy, fine needle aspiration, or core needle biopsy.

In a surgical biopsy, the radiologist locates the abnormality on a mammogram (or sonogram) just prior to surgery. Using the mammogram as a guide, the radiologist inserts a fine needle or wire so the tip rests in the suspect area, typically, an area of microcalcifications. The needle is anchored with gauze bandage, and a second mammogram is taken to confirm that the needle is on target.

The woman, along with her mammograms, goes to the operating room, where the surgeon locates and cuts out the needle-targeted area. The more precisely the needle is placed; the less tissue needs to be removed.

- *Stereotactic localization biopsy* is a newer approach that relies on a three-dimensional x-ray to guide the needle biopsy of a nonpalpable mass. With one type of equipment, the patient lies face down on an examining table with a hole in it that allows the breast to hang through: the x-ray machine and the maneuverable needle "gun" are set up underneath. Alternatively, specialized stereotatic equipment can be attached to a standard mammography machine.

The breast is x-rayed from two different angles and a computer

Early Diagnosis and Treatment Can Save Your Life

plots the exact position of the suspicious area. (Because only small area of the breast is exposed to the radiation, the doses are not similar to those from standard mammography.) Once the target is clearly identified, the radiologist positions the gun and advances the biopsy needle into the lesion.

A woman facing biopsy has a broader range of options. No single solution is right for everyone. Each woman should consult with her doctors and her family, weigh the alternatives, and decide what approach is appropriate. Being involved in the decision-making process can give a woman control over the things that affect her body and her life.

Early Diagnosis and Treatment Can Save Your Life

13
Breast Cancer Treatment Options

Before you consider your treatment options, you will need a team of medical experts who will provide you with enough information and support to make your decision-making process easier. No one doctor can provide you with all the services you may need.

There are a number of treatment options available to you. Before you decide which is the best and the most realistic option, whatever you do, please make sure you do your homework, i.e., research, ask questions of the doctors, ask women who have gone through similar situations, and ask questions of anyone who you feel can offer some advice on helping you to make rational and informed decisions.

YOUR TREATMENT TEAM

If your lump does contain cancer cells, you will need a team of medical experts. No one doctor is able to provide all the services you may need. Here are some of the experts you may need.

- Anesthesiologist: a doctor who gives medications that keep you comfortable during surgery.
- Clinical Nurse Specialist: nurses with special training who can help answer questions and provide information on resources and support services.
- Oncologist: a doctor who uses chemotherapy or hormone therapy to treat cancer.
- Pathologist: a doctor who examines tissue and cells under a microscope to decide if they are normal or cancerous.
- Physical Therapist: a medical professional who teaches exercises that help restore arm and shoulder movements after surgery.
- Plastic Surgeon: a doctor who can rebuild (reconstruct) your breasts.
- Radiation Oncologist: a doctor who uses radiation therapy to treat cancer.
- Radiologist: a doctor who reads mammograms and performs other tests, such as x-rays or ultrasound.
- Social Worker: a professional who can talk with you about your emotional or physical needs.
- Surgeon: a doctor who performs biopsies and other surgical procedures such as the removal of your lump (lumpectomy) or your breast (mastectomy).

If breast cancer is diagnosed, first the breast(s) where the tumor was discovered must be treated. The next priority is to decide whether and how the rest of a patient's body should be treated if there is a strong suspicion the cancer might have spread beyond the breast. Surgery, whether or not followed by radiation therapy, is "primary" local treatment. Depending on the diagnosis, "adjuvant" therapy may be necessary. Adjuvant therapy treatments are given in addition to the primary

Early Diagnosis and Treatment Can Save Your Life

therapy to destroy any cancer cells left behind in the breast or in distant places in a woman's body. This is the purpose of treatment by chemotherapy and "endocrine" (hormonal) therapy.

Decisions to be made start with whether the breast can or should be spared, or whether it would be safer to remove all the breast tissue in a mastectomy procedure. If the breast is to be preserved, then it needs to be decided whether radiation therapy should follow. The next decision is whether or not adjuvant therapy is needed and, if it is, what kind would be best. The surgeon will make recommendations based on what has been learned over many years from results of studying treatment alternatives used by thousands of doctors with tens of thousands of patients in carefully controlled clinical trials. It is also important that the doctor take your particular situation/circumstances under consideration when determining your treatment option.

PRIMARY TREATMENT ALTERNATIVES

"Primary" treatment will be either a mastectomy of some kind, or partial surgery to remove just the tumor (lumpectomy). In either case, some axillary lymph nodes will also be removed for staging purposes. (The lymph nodes are small masses of bean-shaped tissue, located along the lymphatic system, that removes waste and fluids from lymph and acts as filters of impurities in the body). A lumpectomy is usually followed by high-dose x-ray radiation to the preserved breast.

Lumpectomy The lump and a border of surrounding tissue are removed. A few of the lymph nodes in the armpit will probably also be taken out and a biopsy done to see if the cancer has spread there. Even if no cancer is found in the lymph nodes, lumpectomy is always followed by several weeks of radiation therapy. Lumpectomy is usually done for smaller tumors (less than 4 centimeters, or about 1.6 inches). Lumpectomy is not recommended for women with large tumors, especially those with small breasts. The difference in the size of the breast after surgery would be very noticeable and there could be a more even match by having a mastectomy followed by reconstruction.

Early Diagnosis and Treatment Can Save Your Life

Partial or Segmental Mastectomy The tumor and up to one-quarter of the breast tissue are removed. All or just some of the lymph nodes in the armpit are also taken out and radiation therapy usually follows.

Simple or Total Mastectomy The entire breast is removed. For very early cancers, this is often the only treatment needed. In other cases, radiation therapy will follow. Sometimes a few lymph nodes are taken out.

Modified Radical Mastectomy (Total Mastectomy with Axillary Dissection)
The entire breast, the underarm lymph nodes, and the lining over the chest muscles, but not the muscles themselves, are removed. If the woman is at high risk of having the breast cancer return, radiation therapy will also be advised. A woman planning to have breast reconstruction after a modified radical mastectomy should have a surgeon consult with the plastic surgeon before the mastectomy. The way the skin is cut to remove the breast depends on where the tumor is and the method used by the surgeon. Having the skin cut from side to side, rather than from top to bottom of the breast, may allow a woman to wear lower necklines after reconstruction.

Radical Mastectomy This is also known as the Halsted Radical, after its originator, Dr. William Halsted, a Baltimore surgeon practicing around the turn of the century. The breast, the lymph nodes in the armpit, and the chest muscles under the breast are all removed. Afterwards, a woman may feel a loss of strength in the arm on the same side where the breast was removed, and have numbness and swelling in the arm. While this surgery results in greater changes to a woman's body, it is still the treatment of choice for those whose cancers are attached to the chest wall.

Prophylactic Mastectomy Women at very high risk of breast cancer may elect prophylactic (preventive) mastectomy. This is an operation in which one or both breasts are removed before there is a known breast cancer. Recent studies have reported a greater than 90% reduction in risk of breast cancer in high-risk women with family history who received prophylactic mastectomy.

Early Diagnosis and Treatment Can Save Your Life

Subsequent studies confirmed the benefit of prophylactic mastectomy in genetically susceptible women, i.e., women with BRCA1 and BRCA 2 mutations. While the operation reduces the risk of breast cancer, it does not guarantee that cancer won't develop in the small amount of breast tissue remaining after the operation. A woman considering this operation should discuss these considerations carefully with her doctor. A second opinion is strongly recommended.

Lymph Node Surgery Whether a woman has a mastectomy or a lumpectomy for invasive cancer, she and her doctor usually need to know if the cancer has spread to the lymph nodes. If the lymph nodes are affected, it increases the likelihood that cancer cells have spread (*metastasized*) through the bloodstream to other parts of the body. Women with pure ductal carcinoma in situ or pure lobular carcinoma in situ do not need lymph node testing.

Surgery is the only way to accurately determine if the cancer has spread to the lymph nodes. This usually means removing some or all of the lymph nodes in the armpit. Usually 10 to 20 lymph nodes in the armpit are removed. This operation is called an axillary lymph node dissection.

RADIATION THERAPY

The goal of radiation therapy is to destroy cancer cells by stopping their ability to divide, while causing the least amount of damage possible to other cells. In treating breast cancer, radiation is usually used along with a lumpectomy or segmental mastectomy. More and more women have chosen to have lumpectomies and radiation, rather than having the entire breast removed. Studies have shown that for women with small tumors that have not spread outside the breast, lumpectomy plus radiation produce as good results as operations that remove more of the breast.

Early Diagnosis and Treatment Can Save Your Life

Radiation is usually not needed after a mastectomy although it may be given to some women at high risk of having breast cancer recur. For women with advanced cancers, radiation may be used to help make the tumor smaller and easier to remove by surgery, or to help relieve pain caused by the spread of cancer into the bones.

The radiation can be given by a machine (external beam radiation) or by small radioactive pellets inserted in the breast through thin tubes. These implanted pellets remain in place three to four days, during which time the patient must stay in the hospital and cannot see visitors, because the visitors could be harmed by the small doses of radiation given off by the implants. External beam radiation can cause the skin in the area treated to look and feel sunburned, though this gradually fades into a tanned look. The skin may become thicker and for women receiving radiation after a lumpectomy or partial mastectomy, the breasts may become firmer and smaller. If fluid builds up, however, the breasts may become larger.

CHEMOTHERAPY (ADJUVANT THERAPY)

"Chemo" means chemical and "therapy" means treatment. So, chemotherapy is the use of chemicals to treat disease. Chemotherapy is a systemic therapy, which means it affects the whole body by going through the bloodstream. The purpose of chemotherapy and other systemic treatments is to destroy any cancer cells that may have spread from where the cancer started to another part of the body. It involves using anti-cancer drugs to help control, cure, stop the spread of, slow the growth of, relieve symptoms of, and kill cancer cells.

Chemotherapy is effective against cancer cells because the drugs love to interfere with rapidly dividing cells. The side effects of chemotherapy occur because cancer cells aren't the only rapidly dividing cells in your body. The cells in your blood, mouth, intestinal tract, nose, nails, vagina, and hair are also undergoing constant, rapid division. This means that the chemotherapy is going to affect them also.

Early Diagnosis and Treatment Can Save Your Life

A chemotherapy regimen is usually tailored specifically to the breast cancer patient. When planning a chemotherapy regimen, physicians and patients consider the age, overall health, specific elements of the cancer (e.g., stage, grade) other problems, and past or future treatments. Some chemotherapy drugs are administered orally in the form of pills. Chemotherapy may also be given intramuscularly (injected in the muscle), under the skin, topically (on the skin), or injected locally into the cancer area. It can be given at the hospital outpatient clinic, at the doctor's office, or at home. It can last from 30 minutes or less to more than an hour, depending on the drugs used. In general, chemotherapy for breast cancer patients is typically given in three-to-six month treatment sessions.

The strong drugs used in cancer chemotherapy cause more damage to cancer cells than to normal cells and the doctor must be very careful about how large the dose is and how often it is given. The total amount of drugs given must be enough to kill cancer cells, but not so much as to destroy too many healthy cells. Cells that happen to be in the process of dividing, both the normal and the cancerous ones, are most likely to be destroyed by anti-cancer drugs.

Chemotherapy may be used as the only treatment for breast cancer if the cancer is already widespread at the time of diagnosis and other means of treatment are not considered useful. More commonly, however, chemotherapy is used along with surgery, radiation therapy, or both. For this reason, it is often called "adjuvant" therapy, meaning it assists the primary method of treatment. Adjuvant chemotherapy also seems to be the most useful to women who have not yet reached menopause. Some medical experts believe that all women with breast cancer should have follow-up treatments with chemotherapy, but not all doctors agree. Any woman with breast cancer should discuss with her doctor how chemotherapy might help her and what the side effects might be.

These side effects include nausea, loss of appetite, hair loss (alopecia), increased chance of getting infections, bleeding, anemia, fatigue, mouth

Early Diagnosis and Treatment Can Save Your Life

sores (stomatitis), and changes in the menstrual cycle. Most of these side effects stop once treatment does. Any unexpected side effects should be reported to a doctor.

HIGH-DOSE CHEMOTHERAPY

In breast cancer treatment clinical trials, researchers at the National Cancer Institute and other health institutions are testing high-dose chemotherapy to find out if it is better than standard chemotherapy. They are trying to learn if higher doses of drugs can prevent or delay the spread or return of breast cancer better than standard doses of drugs, and which type of treatment helps patients to live longer.

Patients who receive high doses of chemotherapy are at great risk of suffering life-threatening side effects because the treatment damages bone marrow and they no longer are able to produce needed blood cells. To help repair the damage done by high doses of drugs, the treatment includes peripheral blood stem cell transplantation and/or bone marrow transplantation.

HORMONAL THERAPY (TAMOXIFEN)

Hormonal therapy involves changing the levels of hormones that help the cancer grow. Because this therapy affects the entire body and is used along with other methods of treatment, it is also a systemic and adjuvant treatment. At the time of biopsy, breast cancer cells are also checked to see if growth is swayed by the hormones estrogen and progesterone. If they are, the levels of these hormones may be changed.

Tamoxifen, known by the brand name Nolvadex, is a medication in pill form that interferes with the activity of estrogen (a hormone). Tamoxifen has been used for more than 20 years to treat patients with advanced breast cancer. It is used as adjuvant, or additional, therapy following primary treatment for early stage breast cancer. It is most often prescribed for women who have positive hormone receptors (some cells are nourished by the female hormones, estrogen and progesterone).

Early Diagnosis and Treatment Can Save Your Life

Estrogen promotes the growth of breast cancer cells. Tamoxifen works against the effect of estrogen on these cells. It is often called "anti-estrogen." As a treatment for breast cancer, drug slows or stops the growth of cancer cells that are present in the body. As adjuvant therapy, Tamoxifen helps prevent the original breast cancer from returning and also helps prevent the development of new cancers in the other breast. It can be used with other treatments such as chemotherapy to increase the effectiveness of both.

In general, the side effects of Tamoxifen are similar to some of the symptoms of menopause. The most common side effects are hot flashes and vaginal discharge. Some women experience irregular menstrual periods, headaches, fatigue, nauseas and/or vomiting, vaginal dryness or itching, irritation of the skin around the vagina, and skin rash. As is the case with menopause, not all women who take Tamoxifen have these symptoms. Men who take tamoxifen may experience headaches, nausea, and/or vomiting, skin rash, impotence, or a decrease in sexual interest.

Tamoxifen increases the risk of two types of cancer that can develop in the uterus: endometrial cancer, which arises in the lining of the uterus, and uterine sarcoma, which arises in the muscular wall of the uterus. Like all cancers, endometrial cancer and uterine sarcoma are potentially life threatening. Women who have had a hysterectomy (surgery to remove the uterus) and are taking Tamoxifen are not at increased risk of these cancers.

PERIPHERAL BLOOD STEM CELL TRANSPLANTATION

Peripheral blood stem cell transplantation involves the removal of a certain type of blood cell, called a stem cell, from a patient's blood. Stem cells are immature cells from which all blood cells develop as they are needed. Stem cells are able to divide and form more stem cells (copies of themselves) or they can become fully mature red blood cells (erthrocytes), platelets, and white blood cells (leukocytes).

The removed stem cells are frozen and stored while the patient is treated with high-dose chemotherapy. After chemotherapy ends and the drugs are gone from the body, the stem cells are returned to the patient through a vein. The healthy stem cells can then begin to grow and produce all types of blood cells the patient needs to survive.

BONE MARROW TRANSPLANTATION

Bone marrow is the sponge-like material found inside bones that produces blood cells. Bone marrow transplantation can be used in breast cancer treatment. In this procedure, some of a patient's own healthy bone marrow is removed with a needle before treatment begins. The bone marrow is then frozen and stored while the patient is treated with high-dose chemotherapy. Several days after the treatment ends and the drugs are gone from the body, the healthy bone marrow is given back to the patient through a vein. The healthy bone marrow can then begin to produce blood cells that the patient needs to survive. Peripheral blood stem cells and bone marrow transplantation may be used together as part of high-dose chemotherapy.

COMPLIMENTARY AND ALTERNATIVE MEDICINE (CAM)

Complimentary and alternative medicine, as defined by the National Center for Complementary and Alternative Medicine (NCCAM), is a group of diverse medical and health care systems, practices, and products that are not presently considered to be part of conventional medicine. While some scientific evidence exists regarding some CAM therapies, for most there are key questions that are yet to be answered through well-designed scientific studies—questions such as whether these therapies are safe and whether they work for the disease or medical condition for which they are used.
The list of what is considered to be CAM changes continually, as those therapies that are proven to be safe and effective become adopted into conventional health care and as new approaches to health care emerge. Complementary medicine is used together with conventional medicine. An example of a complementary therapy is using aromatherapy to help lessen a patient's discomfort following surgery. Alternative medicine is used in place of conventional medicine. An example of an alternative therapy is using a

Early Diagnosis and Treatment Can Save Your Life

special diet to treat cancer instead of undergoing surgery, radiation, or chemotherapy that has been recommended by a conventional doctor. <u>Integrative</u> medicine, as defined by NCCM, <u>combines</u> mainstream medical therapies and CAM therapies for which there is some high-quality scientific evidence of safety and effectiveness.

NCCAM classifies CAM therapies into five categories, or domains:

1. Alternative Medical Systems
Alternative medical systems are built upon complete systems of theory and practice. Often, these systems have evolved apart from the earlier than the conventional medical approach used in the United States. Examples of alternative medical systems that have developed in Western cultures include homeopathic medicine and naturopathic medicine. Examples of systems that have developed in non-Western cultures include traditional Chinese medicine and Ayurveda.

2. Mind-Body Interventions
Mind-body medicine uses a variety of techniques designed to enhance the mind's capacity to affect bodily function and symptoms. Some techniques that were considered CAM in the past have become mainstream (for example, patient support groups and cognitive-behavioral therapy). Other mind-body techniques are still considered CAM, including meditation, prayer, mental healing, and therapies that use creative outlets such as art, music, or dance.

3. Biologically Based Therapies
Biologically based therapies in CAM use substances found in nature, such as herbs, foods, and vitamins. Some examples include dietary supplements, herbal products, and the use of other so-called natural but as yet scientifically unproven therapies (for example, using shark cartilage to treat cancer).

4. Manipulative and Body-Based Methods
Manipulative and body-based methods in CAM are based on manipula-

Breast Cancer Treatment Options

tion and/or movement of one or more parts of the body. Some examples include chiropractic or osteopathic manipulation, and massage.

5. Energy Therapies
Energy therapies involve the use of energy fields. They are of two types:

Biofield therapies are intended to affect energy fields that purportedly surround and penetrate the human body. The existence of such fields has not yet been scientifically proven. Some forms of energy therapy manipulate biofields by applying pressure and/or manipulating the body by placing the hands in, or through, these fields. Examples including qi gong, Reiki, and Therapeutic Touch.

Bioelectromagnetic-based therapies involve the unconventional use of electromagnetic fields, such as pulsed fields, magnetic fields, or alternating-current or direct-current fields.

DEFINITION OF TERMS
Acupuncture ("AK-yoo-pungk-cher") is a method of healing developed in China at least 2,000 years ago. Today, acupuncture describes a family of procedures involving stimulation of anatomical points on the body by a variety of techniques. American practices of acupuncture incorporate medical traditions from China, Japan, Korea, and other countries. The acupuncture technique that has been most studied scientifically involves penetrating the skin with thin, solid, metallic needles that are manipulated by the hands or by electrical stimulation.

Aromatherapy ("ah-roam-uh-THER-ah-py") involves the use of essential oils (extracts or essences) form flowers, herbs, and trees to promote health and well-being.

Ayurveda ("ah-yur-VAY-dah") is a CAM alternative medical system that has been practiced primarily in the Indian subcontinent for 5,000 years. Ayurveda includes diet and herbal remedies and emphasizes the use of body, mind, and spirit in disease prevention and treatment.

Early Diagnosis and Treatment Can Save Your Life

Chiropractic ("kie-roh-PRAC-tic") is a CAM alternative medical system. It focuses on the relationship between bodily structure (primarily that of the spine) and function, and how that relationship affects the preservation and restoration of health. Chiropractors use manipulative therapy as an integral treatment tool.

Dietary supplements. Congress defined the term "dietary supplement" in the Dietary Supplement Health and Education Act (DSHEA) of 1994. A dietary supplement is a product (other than tobacco) taken by mouth that contains a "dietary ingredient" intended to supplement the diet. Dietary ingredients may include vitamins, minerals, herbs or other botanicals, amino acids, and substances such as enzymes, organ tissues, and metabolites. Dietary supplements come in many forms, including extracts, concentrates, tablets, capsules, gel caps, liquids, and powers. They have special requirements for labeling. Under DSHEA, dietary supplements are considered foods, not drugs.

Electromagnetic fields (EMF, also called electric and magnetic fields) are invisible lines of force that surround all electrical devices. The Earth also produces EMFs; electric fields are produced when there is thunderstorm activity, and magnetic fields are believed to be produced by electric currents flowing at the Earth's core.

Homeopathic ("home-ee-oh-PATH-ic") **medicine** is a CAM alternative medical system. In homeopathic medicine, there is a belief that "like cures like," meaning that small, highly diluted quantities of medicinal substances are given to cure symptoms, when the same substances given at higher or more concentrated doses would actually cause those symptoms.

Massage ("muh-SAHJ") therapists manipulate muscle and connective tissue to enhance function of those tissues and promote relaxation and well-being.

Naturopathic ("nay-chur-o-PATH-ic") **medicine,** or naturopathy, is a CAM alternative medical system. Naturopathic medicine proposes that there is a healing power in the body that establishes, maintains, and restores health. Practitioners work with the patient with a goal of supporting this power,

Early Diagnosis and Treatment Can Save Your Life

through treatments such as nutrition and lifestyle counseling, dietary supplements, medicinal plant, exercise, homeopathy, and treatments from traditional Chinese medicine.

Osteopathic ("ahs-tee-ohj-PATH-ic") **medicine** is a form of conventional medicine that, in part, emphasizes diseases arising in the musculoskeletal system. There is an underlying belief that all of the body's systems work together, and disturbances in one system may affect function elsewhere in the body. Some osteopathic physicians practice osteopathic manipulation, a full-body system of hands-on techniques to alleviate pain, restore function, and promote health and well-being.

Qi gong ("chee-GUNG") is a component of traditional Chinese medicine that combines movement, meditation, and regulation of breathing to enhance the flow of qi (an ancient term given to what is believed to be vital energy) in the body, improve blood circulation, and enhance immune function.

Reiki ("RAY-kee") is a Japanese word representing Universal Life Energy. Reiki is based on the belief that when spiritual energy is channeled through a Reiki practitioner, the patient's spirit is healed, which in turn heals the physical body.

Therapeutic Touch is derived from an ancient technique called laying-on-of hands. It is based on the premise that it is the healing force of the therapist that affects the patient's recovery; healing is promoted when the body's energies are in balance; and, by passing their hands over the patient, healers can identify energy imbalances.

Early Diagnosis and Treatment Can Save Your Life

Traditional Chinese Medicine (TCM) is the current name for an ancient system of health care from China. TCM is based on a concept of balanced qi (pronounced "chee"), or vital energy, that is believed to flow throughout the body. Qi is proposed to regulate a person's spiritual, emotional, mental, and physical balance and to be influenced by the opposing forces of yin (negative energy) and yang (positive energy). Disease is proposed to result from the flow of qi being disrupted and yin and yang becoming imbalanced. Among the components of TCM are herbal and nutritional therapy, restorative physical exercises, meditation, acupuncture, and remedial massage.

CLINICAL TRIALS

Clinical trials are scientific studies of new treatments or combinations of treatments. Each trial is designed to answer a specific question about treatment methods. In a clinical trial, researchers compare standard or proven therapy with a new therapy that may turn out to be better. Patients who agree to be a part of a clinical trial are by chance (randomly) assigned to receive either the standard or the new treatment. Random assignment ensures scientific accuracy of the results. Neither you nor your physician can choose the group you will be in during a clinical trial. The patient's progress is followed and results are compared.

A new treatment is normally studied in three phases of clinical trails before it is eligible for approval by the FDA.

Phase I clinical trials: The purpose of a Phase I study is to find the best way to give a new treatment and how much of it can be given safely. The treatment has been well tested in laboratory and animal studies, but the side effects are not completely known. The main purpose of a Phase I study is to test the safety of the drug.

Phase II clinical trials: These are designed to see if the drug works. Patients are usually given the highest dose that doesn't cause severe side

Early Diagnosis and Treatment Can Save Your Life

effects (determined from the Phase I study) and watched closely for an effect on the cancer. The doctor will also look for side effects.

Phase III clinical trials: Phase III studies involve large numbers of patients. One group (the control group) will receive the standard (most accepted) treatment. The other group will receive the new treatment. The study will be stopped if the side effects of the new treatment are to severe or if one group has had much better results that the others.

If you are in a clinical trial, you will have a team of experts taking care of you and monitoring your progress very carefully. The study is designed to pay close attention to you. The ACS currently has a clinical trials matching service. For questions contact the ACS at 800-303-5691.

GENE TESTING FOR BREAST CANCER SUSCEPTIBILITY

A breast cell progresses from normal to cancerous through a series of several distinct changes, each one controlled by a different gene or set of genes. Researchers have precisely located the BRCA1 and BRCA2 genes, key regions within a woman's chromosomes that control cell growth in breast tissue. A woman can inherit a mutation, an alteration in these genes that are essential for normal growth of breast cells. This inherited change may put her at greater risk for eventually developing breast cancer. The identification of genetic changes in BRCA1 and BRCA2 makes a gene test possible.

Scientists estimate that alterations in the BRCA1 and BRCA2 genes may be responsible for about 5 to 10 percent of all the cases of breast cancer and for about 25 percent of the cases in women under the age of 30. BRCA1 mutation testing is primarily done in certain families whose members are inclined to develop breast cancer at an early age because of an inherited change. Special counseling programs occur before and after the testing to inform women about the possible consequences of

Early Diagnosis and Treatment Can Save Your Life

receiving test results. It is hoped that these genetic tests may one day enable scientists to delay or prevent breast cancer in high-risk families. Positive results may enable careful monitoring when appropriate; negative results may reassure those women in high-risk families who are at no greater than average risk for breast cancer.

In addition to BRCA1 and BRCA2, other genes and the proteins they control may be involved in breast cancer, and much more needs to be learned about the risk associated with particular genetic alterations.

LYMPHEDEMA

A problem that may arise after treatment is swelling of the arm on the side of the mastectomy. Called lymphedema, this condition is caused by the loss of underarm lymph nodes and their connecting vessels. Because the lymph nodes have been removed, circulation of lymph fluid is slowed, making it harder for your body to fight infection. You should take special care of your arm to prevent infection.

No one can predict which patient will develop this condition or when. Lymphedema can develop just after surgery, months, or even years later. Most women, however, do not have serious lymphedema. With care, patients can take steps to help avoid lymphedema, or at least keep it under control. Talk to your doctor for more details. Among the steps to take to help avoid lymphedema:

- Avoid having blood drawn from or IVs inserted into the arm on the side of the lymph node surgery.
- Do not allow a blood pressure cuff to be placed on that arm. If you are in the hospital, tell all health care workers about your arm.
- If your arm or hand feels tight of swollen, don't ignore it. Tell your doctor immediately.
- If needed, wear a well-fitted compression sleeve on the arm. Your doctor can provide you with this.
- Wear gloves when gardening or doing other things that are likely to lead to cuts.

Early Diagnosis and Treatment Can Save Your Life

FOLLOW-UP AND TREATMENT FOR BREAST CANCER THAT RECURS

Medical Care
Women who have been treated for breast cancer should continue to receive follow-up examinations throughout their lifetimes, since it is possible that breast cancer may return even 30 years after it is first found. A woman should ask her doctor how often these follow-up examinations should be done. Generally, it depends on the type and stage of breast cancer, the type of treatment, and the risk of the cancer recurring.

Your relationship with your health care team is for life. If you move, be sure to take your medical records with you or have them sent to your new doctor. If you need a recommendation for a new doctor, consult your current one or get a referral from the county medical association.

Most doctors agree that during the first year, you should make a follow-up visit every two to three months. In following years, you should set up a schedule of visits with your treatment team as they recommend. Be aware of any pain in your shoulder, hip, lower back, or pelvis. Also note any unusual breast ache or pain that does not come and go with your menstrual cycle. You should be sure to report immediately any such changes to your doctor.

The most important part of your follow-up care is up to you. Have a mammogram and breast exam by your doctor every year and do monthly breast self-exams.

Breast Self-Exams After Breast Surgery
It is very important that you keep doing regular breast self-exam on both breasts, including the surgical area. Feel gently, carefully, and thoroughly. If you find something you think is abnormal, contact your doctor. Be sure to examine the sides of the chest, armpits, and particularly the scar area.

Early Diagnosis and Treatment Can Save Your Life

Because tissue changes do occur after surgery, you will have to learn from your doctor what is normal for you. Regular checkups will teach you what is normal for your body and give you confidence in your self-examination.

Nutrition and Lifestyle

Two factors believed to increase the risk of breast cancer are obesity and a high-fat diet. A diet that includes large amount of foods high in fat, especially animal fat, can contribute to excessive weight gain. Eating foods low in fat will not only contribute to weight loss, but will also help improve your overall health.

Other steps you can take to get to and/or maintain a healthy weight are to limit your consumption of sugary foods, fast foods, caffeine, and alcoholic beverages. You can add foods that are high in fiber and lower in calories, such as fruits, vegetables, and whole grains. Exercise is another way to help reduce your weight and to improve your overall health.

OPTIONS AFTER TREATMENT

Breast Prosthesis

After a mastectomy, women have the option of either wearing a prosthesis (artificial breast form) or having breast reconstruction to restore the natural shape and contour of the breast. The choice is a personal one based on your individual needs, desires, lifestyle, and physical or medical limitations. Each woman is different. You should take the time you need to make the choice that is right for you. Try not to be influenced by what someone else thinks is best for you. Make your own decision.

Temporary Prosthesis

If you would like some contour under your clothes or nightgown, this breast form may be pinned inside your clothes or worn inside a loose-fitting bra. It may be hand washed, then placed inside the foot of a old stocking and placed in the dryer. You may need to reshape it to regain the contour you need.

Early Diagnosis and Treatment Can Save Your Life

If the color of your breast form is not dark enough, try dipping it in strong coffee or tea to get the desired shade. If necessary you can use Rit dye (light or dark brown). The dye takes very quickly so only dip the form in the solution two or three times and then rinse under cold water.

Permanent Prostheses
Once your incision is completely healed and your doctor has given permission, you can begin to shop for a permanent prosthesis or breast form. There is a wide range of styles and types available. Most of them feel the same and weigh the same as normal breast tissue.

When you shop for a prosthesis, wear a form-fitting garment such as a knit dress that will drape nicely and give you a very clear look at the shape and contour of your breast. Try the prosthesis on in a comfortable, supporting bra. Be sure the form matches as closely as possible to the shape of your other breast from the sides, top, bottom, and front. You should always be fitted by a trained and experienced fitter.

Ask your doctor to write a prescription for your prosthesis and for any special bras to receive insurance reimbursement. The ACS office nearest you may be able to give you a list of stores that carry and fit prostheses.

If you are unable or do not want to purchase a prosthesis, you can make your own. Using polyester or Dacron fluff, which can be obtained at craft or sewing centers, make a form to fit your contour. The fluff can be placed in a cover that is the shape of your bra cup. To weight the form, use drapery weights or fishing sinkers interspersed in the fluff. The larger your other breast, the more important it is to buy or make a weighted form. The weights of your natural breast and the prosthesis need to be balanced for better posture and comfort.

Early Diagnosis and Treatment Can Save Your Life

BREAST IMPLANTS

The oldest and simplest method of reconstructing the breast is to create a mound with a synthetic implant. The surgeon inserts the implant through the mastectomy incision and under the pectoralis major (chest) muscle. Occasionally, the surgeon may insert the implant through a new incision on the side of the breast nearest the armpit.

Implants that differ in both size and shape are available. Each type has advantages and disadvantages. From an appearance point of view, women with small to medium, rounded breasts have the best results with implants matching the opposite breasts.

Types of Implants

There is still some controversy about the safety of silicone gel implants. Many women prefer them to saline-filled implants because the silicone feels more like breast tissue, and the gel shifts with movement more naturally. However, if a leak occurs, saline is absorbed into the body and is harmless. There has been a question whether silicone can trigger certain connective tissue and auto immune conditions (diseases in which the body's immune system attacks normal tissues). Studies completed thus far have failed to show an increased risk of autoimmune disease among women with silicone implants.

Regardless of the type of implant, the actual surgery to insert the implant is relatively simple. When done at the time of a mastectomy, the reconstruction adds only about a half hour to an hour to the surgery. There are drains in place, and recovery time is longer due to the additional surgery, but the care afterward is the same as for mastectomy alone. Delayed reconstruction requires about an hour and a half. Drains are not routine, and recovery is much quicker than it is after immediate reconstruction because the mastectomy wound has already healed.

The surgeon usually inserts a temporary tissue expander under the pectoralis muscle to stretch the muscle and the skin over the chest wall. The tissue expander is a silicone envelope with a valve-like opening or port through which a small amount of saline is injected. Every week or two for one to three months saline is injected until the expander is inflated to a size slightly larger than the implant will be. This stretching is painless just like the stretching of a abdomen that occurs with pregnancy.

Once the tissues are able to accommodate an implant and allow for a natural droop of the breasts, the surgeon will replace the expander with a permanent implant. This is a 30-minute operation that can be done on an outpatient basis. Usually general anesthesia is used, but no overnight stay is required.

Complications and side effects of implants.
As with any surgery, there is a risk of postoperative complications such as infection, seroma (accumulation of fluid in the surgical wound), and bleeding. In the case of reconstruction, these problems also include a loss of sensation in the breast; movement of the implant; breast asymmetry, or difference in the size and/or shape of the breasts; and extrusion, in which the implant begins to push out through the healing incision. The most common complication is a phenomenon known as capsular contraction, in which the pocket of scar tissue that forms around the implant becomes abnormally hard and contracts over the implant, causing the reconstructed breast to be misshapen.

Lattissimus dorsi flap.
If there is not enough skin to cover the implant, if the muscle over the chest wall has been removed, or if the skin has been so damaged by radiation that it cannot be stretched, the surgeon will remove a fan-shaped section of muscle and skin from the back attached to a portion of tissue, called a pedicle. The pedicle remains intact and contains the blood supply of the flap. This latissimus dorsi flap, which is named for the back muscle from which it comes, is tunneled under the skin and pulled out through an opening in the chest. It is then sutured in place over the mastectomy site. The surgeon then places an implant under the muscle to complete the reconstruction.

The latissimus dorsi flap procedure is obviously a much more complicated operation than an implant insertion. There is a scar on the woman's back, and there is a potential for shoulder problems because a portion of the muscle governing range of motion to the shoulder has been removed. There is about a two percent risk that a portion of the flap will not heal properly, and another operation may be necessary. However, this procedure usually creates a better result than when an implant is used alone, particularly in women with large breasts, or in women after radiation.

BREAST RECONSTRUCTION

Breast reconstruction is a surgical procedure which attempts to restore in the woman's body the contour of the breast that was removed. Breast reconstruction can be successfully performed immediately, at the same time as mastectomy, or some time later. Most physicians agree that breast reconstruction is safe, and does not interfere with follow-up care after surgery such as regular mammograms and breast self-examination. Women seek breast reconstruction for a number of reasons, including:

- The comfort and convenience of not having to wear a prosthesis.
- An enhanced sense of sexual attractiveness.
- More variety in the type and style of clothing that can be worn.
- A reduced preoccupation with breast cancer.
- A restored sense of freedom and a feeling of being physically renewed.

Autologous Reconstruction of the Breasts

Several techniques can be used to reconstruct the breast using the patient's own tissue. A quantity of fatty tissue and small amount of muscle may be transplanted from the abdomen, back or buttocks. This is possible only if the patient has enough soft tissue mass in those areas. If a woman is very slender and lacks sufficient fatty tissue, an implant can be used. The most common technique, the TRAM flap, carries its own blood supply.

Early Diagnosis and Treatment Can Save Your Life

Another method, the free flap, requires meticulous and difficult microsurgery to connect tiny blood vessels in the flap to those in the chest wall.

TRAM Flap

The TRAM (Transverse Rectus Abdominous Muscle) flap uses tissue taken from the woman's abdomen. The surgery is complicated and time-consuming, adding many hours to a mastectomy operation when the reconstruction is immediate.

A section of skin, underlying fat, and a portion of abdominal muscle is excised, leaving one or two pedicles of tissue with the natural blood supply. The flap is tunneled under the abdominal wall to the chest and rotated to fit the mastectomy wound. The edges of the breast incision are sutured to the flap.

Along with creating a breast with natural texture, the technique also gives the stomach a flatter appearance. However, some doctors caution against thinking of this as a tummy tuck, as there are side effects not normally associated with the cosmetic procedure. (For instance, some women experience abdominal weakness, sometimes to the point of being unable to do a sit-up). There is also an increased risk of developing an abdominal hernia (bulging of internal tissues through an area of weakness in the abdominal muscles and connective tissues). The TRAM flap can be sculpted to create a shape to match the other breast instead of just the typical round shape of an implant.

The TRAM flap procedure is major surgery that requires a week in the hospital and another four to six weeks or longer of recovery at home. Women who smoke cannot have this operation. They are likely to develop healing problems because smoking causes deterioration of the blood vessels. Although this operation is performed more than tissue expanders for women after radiation, it does have a higher rate of complications. In these women, fresh, unirradiated tissue is brought into the breast area. Women with abdominal scars or women without enough abdominal fat are not candidates for this surgery.

Early Diagnosis and Treatment Can Save Your Life

Free Flap
This is sometimes called a free TRAM because an island of fat and skin is removed from the abdomen. However, rather than leaving a pedicle attached to a blood supply, the entire island is cut "free" and stitched in place to the mastectomy wound. A surgeon who specializes in microsurgery attaches the blood vessels supplying the flap to those in the chest wall. Since it's not necessary to remove as much muscle from the abdomen, the side effects of the TRAM muscle removal, including abdominal hernia, should be avoided.

A free flap graft can also be made from the soft tissue, muscle and skin of the buttocks. The gluteal free flap is performed when other options are not possible. It may cause hip problems; the sciatic nerve may become injured causing leg pain, numbness, and weakness, and it is technically more difficult to accomplish than the free TRAM procedure.

Complications
Autologous breast reconstruction is major surgery that can require many hours in the operating room. The immediate complications are those associated with any operation, such as infection, formation of blood clots in the legs (which is why you will be encouraged to move about in bed after surgery and get out of bed the next day), and accumulation of blood and/or fluid in the breasts or donor site that must be drained.

Much more likely, though still not common, are complications in healing. If the blood supply is not adequate, the skin over the reconstructed breast may not heal properly and will die, requiring another operation to replace it. Sometimes, too, fatty tissue degenerates and causes a thickening that can be painful and feels similar to a lump or tumor, which can be very frightening. The surgeon will take a biopsy of the thickening to check for cancer cells. Fluid or blood may continue to accumulate and must be withdrawn through a needle or the surgeon may insert a drain that allows the liquid to exit the body.

Early Diagnosis and Treatment Can Save Your Life

Nipple/Areola Reconstruction

In order to give the breast a realistic appearance, many women choose to have the nipple and surrounding areola reconstructed also. There are several techniques used to accomplish this, but usually tissue from heavier skin from the upper inner thigh is used. (Labial tissue is not used.) Some tissue from just under the skin can create nipple projection. When healing is complete, the areola can be tattooed with the flesh-colored pigment. This refinement procedure is most often done after the reconstructed breast has healed completely.

Early Diagnosis and Treatment Can Save Your Life

14

Ask Questions... Then Ask More Questions

I can't stress enough the importance of asking questions. It allows you to take an active role in decisions that affect you, thereby making you the best advocate for your health care. I know from personal experience that questioning your doctor can be uncomfortable, maybe even scary, but don't feel intimidated by the doctors and don't let them make you feel that you don't have a right to question his or her advice and recommendations. No question is off limits. If you think about it, ask it. If you feel that your question is off base, tactfully find a way to ask your doctor or write your doctor a letter. Just make sure that your questions are answered and that you fully understand their answers. You'll be surprised at the results you'll get if you understand what's going on with your body and the way the doctors treat you. Don't relinquish all your power to the doctors and let them make decisions for you. Any health issue, not only breast cancer, should be a joint venture between doctor and patient.

Many people feel intimidated in the doctor's office because they're not sure what questions to ask, or forget their questions when they are ready to ask them. Before your doctor's appointment, get a pen, notepad, and have a list of questions that you want to ask the doctor. (If you feel that you need someone to accompany you, you have every right to bring someone.)

If your doctor can't, won't, or doesn't satisfy your requests, then you go see another, and another, and another, until all your questions and concerns have been addressed and resolved.

Most importantly, get a doctor you feel comfortable with and one who will listen to you.

Early Diagnosis and Treatment Can Save Your Life

QUESTIONS TO ASK YOUR DOCTOR ABOUT BREAST CANCER

The following is a series of questions that you might want to ask your doctor. The first is a series of general questions that are for young women wanting to learn about breast cancer. These are followed by more specific questions about mammograms, breast cancer diagnoses, breast biopsy, breast cancer surgery, after-surgery considerations, radiation therapy, chemotherapy, hormone therapy, and breast reconstruction. By doing your homework you will know if the answer the doctor gives is the best answer for you. This will also help you become proactive in your health care.

General Questions About Breast Cancer

What factors increase breast cancer risk in younger women?
Simply getting older and being a woman puts every woman at risk. However, certain factors have been identified which increase the odds:

Family History. A woman is considered at higher risk for breast cancer if she has a mother, sister or daughter who has been diagnosed with breast cancer. Five percent of all breast cancer patients, but as many as 25 percent of women diagnosed at age 35 or younger, are believed to carry the breast cancer gene, BRCA1. A carrier of BRCAI has an 85 percent lifetime chance of developing breast cancer.

Atypical Hyperplasia. This type of noncancerous breast disease is characterized by a growth of abnormal cells within the ducts. Premenopausal women with a biopsy confirmed diagnosis of atypical hyperplasia are at increased risk for developing invasive breast cancer.

Pregnancy. A woman who has her first child after age 30 or who has no children has a *slightly* increased lifetime risk of breast cancer.

Menstrual History. Women who began menstruating before age 12 or completed menopause after age 55 also have a slightly increased risk.

Early Diagnosis and Treatment Can Save Your Life

Oral Contraceptives. Although the link between the birth control pill and breast cancer remains unresolved, the most recently published report showed a slight increased risk for women currently using the pill or who have used oral contraceptives in the past ten years. However, for those women who have not used the pill for ten or more years, there is no evidence of increased risk.

Alcohol. A study published in June 1995 found an increased incidence of breast cancer in women who consumed one to two drinks or more a day. This study confirmed the findings of other studies, which have linked alcohol with increased risk, but further studies are still under way.

Radiation Therapy for Hodgkin's Disease. Young women successfully treated for malignant lymphomas, including Hodgkin's disease, with radiation to nodal areas of the upper torso have an increased risk of developing breast cancer ten years after their last radiation treatment.

Diet, Exercise, and Environment. The role that diet, exercise, and environmental factors might play in the development of breast cancer is still unknown and is under investigation. Studies have been contradictory in all of these areas. A lowfat, high fiber diet may protect against many diseases, and at least one study has shown that physically active women have a reduced risk of breast cancer.

Does breast size affect breast cancer risk?
No. There is no correlation between breast size and cancer risk.

Does smoking cause breast cancer?
Although the majority of studies have not found that smoking causes breast cancer, one recent study suggests there may be a link, and some studies have shown that smoking decreases a woman's chance of surviving breast cancer once diagnosed. The carcinogenic effect of smoking on most body tissues has been well established, and smoking is the single most preventable cause of disease and death in the United States today.

Early Diagnosis and Treatment Can Save Your Life

What can I do to decrease my chances of developing breast cancer?
The best chance a woman has to fight breast cancer is to find it and treat it early. No one knows what causes breast cancer or how to prevent it. The ACS recommends the following:

- At age 40, begin having annual screening mammograms and continue having them through your 70s.
- Have a nurse or doctor check your breasts every year.
- Examine your breasts every month, and see a doctor if you feel or see any changes.
- Eat a low fat diet, don't smoke, exercise, and drink in moderation, if at all.

Why aren't younger women encouraged to get regular mammograms?
Major medical organizations do not recommend that women under 40 get regular mammograms. Women under age 40 should have a nurse or doctor check their breasts once a year. They should also examine their own breasts every month. A nurse or doctor should evaluate any breast changes. However, if a woman has a family history of pre-menopausal breast cancer, she should talk to her doctor about additional screening, including mammography.

Do young women have a different type of breast cancer than older women?
Younger women are often diagnosed with more advanced cases of breast cancer. This may be due to a delay in diagnosis, in part because young women may not be in a regular screening program. In these women, tumors are larger and their disease is more likely to have spread to the lymph nodes. However, most experts feel that the disease itself is not different in young patients.

Early Diagnosis and Treatment Can Save Your Life

How is breast cancer treated in young women?
Every woman diagnosed with breast cancer decides on the course of her treatment with her physician. Treatment could include a lumpectomy (removal of lump with some surrounding tissue), or a mastectomy (removal of breast). Lumpectomy must be followed by radiation treatment for equal survival benefit. Chemotherapy and/or hormonal therapy are often used in addition to surgery to decrease the chance of reoccurrence. Many young women treated with chemotherapy retain their fertility after treatment is completed. Several studies document safe and successful pregnancies in young breast cancer survivors. A woman considering pregnancy is generally counseled to wait two or more years after treatment, the period in which cancer is most likely to recur.

Does health insurance cover mammography?
Yes, most insurance covers the cost of mammography. Check with your insurance agent or carrier for the specifics of what your plan covers. Medicare covers mammograms. Coverage under Medicaid varies from state to state.

Does the use of hormones to relieve menopausal symptoms cause breast cancer?
Most researchers agree that the use of hormones for contraception or for menopausal symptoms does not increase breast cancer risk.

If a breast lump is painful, is it more likely to be a cancer?
As a breast cancer is developing in the breast, it usually does not cause pain. In the early stages of breast cancer, a woman usually is unaware of any symptoms. But any changes—lumps or pain—should be checked by your health care provider.

Does handling the breasts during lovemaking or by palpation (examination by feeling the tissue) cause breast cancer?
No. Breast cancer is not associated with bumping, bruising, or handling the breasts in any way.

Early Diagnosis and Treatment Can Save Your Life

What if I'm afraid I will find a lump doing BSE?
It is natural for a woman to feel apprehensive when she first begins routine self-examination. Practicing breast self-examination regularly can help decrease this apprehension. And by doing so, you become familiar with your breasts and able to detect any changes.

What about treatment for early breast cancer?
There are more treatment options when the cancer is small. In many cases, the breast may be saved. If you are told you have breast cancer, you should talk with your health care provider about your treatment options. Appropriate treatment is recommended for the individual patient depending upon the stage of the cancer at the time it is detected. You should be told of the advantages and impact the treatment will have on your quality of life.

What are my chances of surviving if I get breast cancer?
Survival depends primarily on the stage of the disease at the time it is detected. Early detection is the key and that means following the American Cancer Society guidelines for mammography, clinical examination, and monthly self-exam.

Am I at an increased risk for breast cancer if I have breast cysts?
Only a very small number of women with fibrocystic breasts have a slightly increased risk of developing breast cancer, and those women can be identified by a pathologist's examination of breast tissue.

How can I increase my confidence in doing BSE?
The first step in increasing confidence is being comfortable with your body. The next step is to learn how to perform BSE correctly. By following the guidelines for early detection, every woman can reduce her fear of hidden breast cancers. Women improve their ability to feel changes in their breasts each time they do self-examination. Monthly self-examination combined with mammography and clinical examination provides every woman with the opportunity for early detection.

Early Diagnosis and Treatment Can Save Your Life

Does mammography cause breast cancer?
No. The benefits of early detection are clear and the risk of breast cancer from radiation is so low as to be negligible. Recent improvements in mammography equipment and technique have greatly lowered the amount of radiation needed to produce a high-quality image of the breast tissue. Women should be reassured that the very low levels of radiation involved are no cause for concern.

Is mammography alone a certain way of detecting breast cancer?
No, the American Cancer Society recommends using all three exams—clinical breast exam, mammography, and BSE—as the best possible approach to detecting breast cancer. However, mammography is the single best way to detect breast cancer early.

How does a health care provider evaluate a breast lump?
When a woman finds a lump, she should go to her health care provider without delay. Her health care provider will usually examine both breasts and decide if a lump or other suspicious change needs further investigation. A mammogram may be ordered. And the health care provider may remove the lump through surgery or use a needle to remove tissue. The pathologist who examines the sample of breast tissue under a microscope can only make the final diagnosis of cancer.

I fear my health care provider will consider my breast symptoms trivial. What can I do about this?
It is important that you select a health care provider with whom you are comfortable and can discuss your concerns. Breast changes are not trivial and should be examined carefully by a health care provider. The health care provider may decide that a breast lump or change does not require immediate treatment. Frequent followup exams may be recommended. The coordinated effort of each woman and her health care provider is the best means for controlling breast cancer.

Early Diagnosis and Treatment Can Save Your Life

Ask Questions...Then Ask More Questions

Do you think it will be too painful to get a mammogram?
Some women do experience discomfort, but usually it is brief. Again, the positive aspects of getting a mammogram outweigh the negative. If menstruating, a woman should wait and get a mammogram after her period, when her breasts are less likely to be tender.

I'm afraid that being partially undressed in front of a stranger would make me feel uncomfortable and keep me from getting a mammogram. What should I do?
Mammography technicians are aware that this is an awkward situation for many women and are usually very sympathetic and understanding. If you feel uncomfortable, tell the mammography technician how you feel and that this is your first mammogram. Most mammograms are given by a woman technician, and you are given a cover up to wear, except during the mammogram. Also, a mammogram does not take long. You can request that you be seen by a female technician.

My doctor has never told me to get a mammogram, so why should I?
As a woman grows older, her chance of having breast cancer increases. You were probably seeing your health care provider for another reason, and just didn't think about it. Your health is your responsibility. Initiate the conversation with your physician and request a mammogram.

Questions Involving The Mammography Process

Where can I get a mammogram?

What do I do to prepare for a mammogram?

Does the FDA certify the mammogram facility?

How long will it take to receive the report on the mammogram? Can I discuss my x-ray with the radiologist?

How much will the mammogram cost?

Early Diagnosis and Treatment Can Save Your Life

Questions To Ask Your Doctor If You Discover A Lump

Will you refer me to a mammography facility for a mammogram?

Does the mammogram facility meet quality standards?

Can this lump be aspirated (fluid or cells removed with a needle)?

Will you refer me to a doctor who specializes in breast problems for further tests and/or treatment?

Do you use machines specifically designed for mammography?
(**Note:** These are called "dedicated" mammography machines. Do not choose a facility that uses a machine that also takes xrays of the bones and other parts of the body.)

Is the person who provides the mammogram a registered technologist?

Is the radiologist who reads the mammograms specially trained to do so?

Does the facility provide mammograms as part of its regular practice?
(**Note:** The American College of Radiology suggests choosing a facility that performs at least ten mammograms per week.)

Is the mammography machine calibrated at least once a year?

Is there anything I should do to prepare for my mammogram?

What will the mammogram show?

Who gets the report of my mammogram? Can it also be sent to other doctors who treat me?

How long will it take to receive the mammography report?

What are the next steps if my mammogram finds a problem?

Early Diagnosis and Treatment Can Save Your Life

Questions To Ask About Breast Biopsy

If a lump is present, or an abnormal sign appears on a mammogram, there is only one way to know if it is cancer. A surgeon must remove part or all of the suspicious tissue. The specimen must then go to a pathologist, who completes the biopsy and reports whether or not the specimen shows cancer cells. *A lump that can be felt should be biopsied, even if the mammogram is normal.*

Before you agree to a biopsy, you may want to get a second opinion. This way, an additional expert from a hospital or mammography facility will read your mammogram. Your doctor can arrange this for you, or you can have the films sent to the expert you have selected.

What type of biopsy will I have and why?

Will the entire lump be removed or just part of it?

Can the lump be aspirated (the fluid drained or a small number of cells removed) with a needle?

How reliable is a needle biopsy?

How long will the biopsy or aspiration take?

Will I be awake during the biopsy or aspiration and can it be done on an outpatient basis?

If I do have cancer, what other tests should I have?

Will estrogen or progesterone receptor tests be done on the biopsied tissue you remove? What will these tests tell you?

Will other special tests (flow cytometry and other markers for tumor aggressiveness) be done on the tissue?

Early Diagnosis and Treatment Can Save Your Life

Will you do a two-step procedure? (With a two-step procedure, the patient is informed of treatment options after the biopsy results are available. Any further surgery is done as a separate procedure.)

What are the disadvantages of the two-step procedure?

How visible will the scar be?

Are there any after-effects of a biopsy? If so, what are they?

After the biopsy, how soon will I know if I have cancer?

After a biopsy, if cancer is found, how much time can I take to decide what type of treatment to have?

If your biopsy report comes back negative or benign, you do not have cancer. Be sure to:

- Continue seeing your health care provider for routine breast exams.
- Have regular mammograms.
- Continue doing monthly breast selfexams.

Questions To Ask When Breast Cancer Is Diagnosed

What did my biopsy or needle aspiration show?

What kind of breast cancer do I have?

What were the results of my estrogen and progesterone tests? What were the results of the other tests (flow cytometry and other markers of tumor aggressiveness)?

What tests will I have before surgery to see if the cancer has spread to any other organs (liver, lungs, and bones)?

Early Diagnosis and Treatment Can Save Your Life

What are my treatment options? What procedure(s) are you recommending for me and why?

What are the potential risks and benefits of these procedures?

What is your opinion about breast conserving surgery lumpectomy followed by radiation therapy? Am I a candidate for this type of treatment?

Will I need additional treatment with radiation therapy, chemotherapy, and/or hormonal therapy following my surgery? If so, can you refer me to a medical oncologist?

Can breast reconstruction be done at the time of the surgery, as well as later? Would you recommend it for me?

What potential risks and benefits are involved?

If I choose not to have reconstruction, how good are currently available breast prostheses?

How long do I have to make a treatment decision?

What is a clinical trial? Is there a clinical trial that is enrolling patients with my type of breast cancer? If so, how can I learn more?

Could you recommend a breast cancer specialist for a second opinion?

Where will the surgical scar(s) be?

What side effects should I expect after the operation?

How should I expect to feel after the operation?

Early Diagnosis and Treatment Can Save Your Life

Questions To Ask About Radiation Therapy

What year did you (the doctor) complete training in medical oncology?

Why is radiation therapy being recommended?

Do you think that the size, location, and type of breast cancer I have will respond to radiation therapy?

How long will each treatment take? How long will the whole series last?

How soon should treatment begin?

Who will be responsible for my radiation treatments? Who will administer them?

Where will these treatments be done?

Can I come alone or should a friend or relative accompany me?

What side effects should I expect and how long might they last.

What are the risks of this treatment?

What are the precautions or prohibitions during treatment? After treatment (skin creams, lotion, underarm shaving, etc.)?

Can I continue normal activities (work, sex, sports, etc.) during treatment? After treatment?

How often are checkups and tests required after treatment is completed?

How many weeks will I get radiation treatments and how long will each visit be?

Early Diagnosis and Treatment Can Save Your Life

Are there any new therapies available?

Will other therapies be needed?

Questions To Ask About Chemotherapy

How long have you (the doctor) been treating breast cancer with chemotherapy?

Why is chemotherapy indicated in my case?

What is the significance of lymph node involvement?

How many of my lymph nodes are involved?

If my lymph nodes are not involved, should chemotherapy or hormone therapy still be considered?

What drugs will I be taking?

Why have you chosen these particular drugs for me?

What are the drugs supposed to do?

What are the short- and long term risks involved?

What are the possible side effects of this type of chemotherapy? Are they permanent?

Does chemotherapy cause infertility?

Which side effects should I report to the doctor immediately?

How soon should the chemotherapy be started?

Early Diagnosis and Treatment Can Save Your Life

How and where will the chemotherapy be given?

How long will each treatment take? How long will the whole series last?

Can I continue to work, exercise, etc. during these treatments?

Will I need to be admitted to the hospital during the course of my chemotherapy?

Can I come alone for treatments or should a friend or relative accompany me?

Are there other special precautions I should take while on chemotherapy or afterwards?

If I lose my hair, will the cost of a wig be covered by health insurance?

When the treatments are completed, how often will I need to be seen by the oncologist?

Questions To Ask About Breast Reconstruction (For Plastic Surgeon)

Are you (the doctor) a Board certified plastic surgeon?

If so, how long have you been certified?

What type of surgery do you recommend and why?

What are the risks and benefits associated with it?

Can I see photos of women who have had the same type of reconstruction I'm having?

Can I talk with some of your patients about the operation?

Early Diagnosis and Treatment Can Save Your Life

How long will the surgery last?

How long will I be in the hospital? How long is the recovery period after the surgery?

What will the reconstructed breast look and feel like right after surgery? In six months? In a year?

Will I have feeling in the reconstructed breast or nipple?

Is nipple reconstruction done at the same time as the reconstruction? How much will it cost? Is it covered by insurance?

What are the types of reconstructive surgery?

What type is best for me and why?

What chance is there of rejection and/or infection of any implant?

Are there any other risks or side effects to consider?

What can be done if the operation is unsuccessful?

When is the best time for me to have reconstruction—at the same time as the mastectomy? Some time after surgery? After chemotherapy?

If I do not choose reconstruction, what prostheses or breast forms are available?

How many operations are needed? How long a hospital stay is necessary for each?

How much time is needed for recovery after each? Are there any medications to avoid before surgery?

Early Diagnosis and Treatment Can Save Your Life

Is there much pain after surgery? For how long?

Are special bras needed after surgery? Where do I purchase them?

How can I expect the reconstruction to look and feel? How will the reconstructed breast compare in appearance with my healthy breast? Will anything need to be done to the healthy breast?

Will I be able to detect a possible recurrence after reconstructive surgery?

Will my health insurance cover this type of surgery?

Questions To Ask After Breast Surgery

Are there special exercises I should be doing? What type do you recommend? How long should I continue them?

Are there any precautions I should take? (If lymph nodes were removed, should I avoid getting shots in that arm or shaving under that arm?)

When will I be able to get back to my normal routine?

What problems, specifically, should I report to you? If additional therapy is being considered, can you refer me to a Medical Oncologist?

When the additional therapy is completed, who will be responsible for follow-up? How often should I return for an exam? For lab tests or x-rays?

What tests will be done at these times? What will the tests tell us?

Questions To Ask About Hormone Therapy

Which hormones are you recommending for me and why? What are the hormones supposed to do?

Early Diagnosis and Treatment Can Save Your Life

What are the short- and long-term side effects of this hormone treatment?

How soon should the hormone therapy be started? How long will I be taking the hormones?

In what form and how often will the treatment be given?

Will I be given the hormone therapy along with other forms of treatment?

Are the costs of the hormone treatment covered by my health insurance?

<u>Questions You Should Ask About Clinical Trials</u>

What is the purpose of the study, and what kinds of tests are involved?

What does this treatment do, and how long does the treatment last? Can I stop any time I want?

What are the possible side effects and risks?

What is likely to happen in my case with, or without, this new research treatment?

What are my other choices and their advantages and disadvantages?

Who pays for the expenses for my care and treatment during the trial?

If I am harmed as a result of the research, what treatment would I be entitled to?

What type of long-term follow-up care is part of the study?

Has the treatment been used to treat other types of cancers?

The American Cancer Society offers a clinical trials matching service that will help you find a clinical trial that is right for you. You can reach them by calling 800-ACS-2345. You also can get a list of current National Cancer Institute sponsored clinical trials by calling the NCI Cancer Information Service at 800-4-CANCER.

Early Diagnosis and Treatment Can Save Your Life

15

Just For Men

Breast cancer will affect men one way or another: Either someone they love will have it or, in some cases, they will have it themselves. I want to address both issues.

After giving a presentation, a man whose girlfriend had been diagnosed with breast cancer approached me. "Thank you so much for sharing your story," he said. "I really didn't understand what my girlfriend was going through until I heard your story."

Breast cancer is a 'family' disease that attacks the emotions of all those who love you. The feelings of a spouse, significant other or just a male friend are no exception to that rule. The same sense of helplessness that sweeps those fighting the disease also affects the men in their lives who don't know how to help them. The best thing a man can do to support his loved one is to just be emotionally and physically available to them. Aside from dying of this disease, a woman's greatest fear facing this demon is that she will be rejected by the man of her life. Just keep reassuring her of your love and that her fight will be your fight— a "team" battle.

Try to find creative ways to support her. For example, as an act of solidarity, a football player shaved his head when his wife began chemotherapy. It could be something as simple as little notes left or a bouquet of flowers. Deliberate acts of kindness will reassure her she is not alone and she's still considered the same woman you love—with or without a breast.

To prepare yourself, it's important to research the disease and treatment options along with her to better understand the physical and emotional road she faces. It serves a two-fold purpose by demonstrating in action your concern and creating a fully informed partner. Seek out support

Early Diagnosis and Treatment Can Save Your Life

groups and counseling that address your concerns for her and your own fears. Check with your local cancer society which can recommend support groups specifically for men.

Also, let her experience be a reminder to you that breast cancer can invade your body as well. You, too, should initiate breast self exams. More than 1600 men each year thought just like me that this wasn't "their" disease. That changed with a few simple words—"You have breast cancer."

While there continues to be research and outreach on this sorely overlooked segment; a strong message needs to be sent that breast exams be included as a part of men's total health care regimen. Any type of lump, dimpling and/or bleeding of the nipple should be addressed by a doctor immediately. Unfortunately, men (just like some women) tend to discount or ignore the symptoms and wait too long.

Men find that they experience many of the same emotions that women do when diagnosed with breast cancer—anger, resentment, guilt, anxiety, and fear. Some men find it difficult or embarrassing to talk about their breast cancer because it is considered a woman's disease. These are all normal reactions and are part of the process many people go through in trying to come to terms with their illness.

I can't help but wonder if there are more men who suffer in silence from this disease than we know. Men with chiseled bodies, buffed arms, and beautiful chests—men whose bodies betray them as well. Don't let pride, embarrassment, or ignorance cause you to lose your life.

Early Diagnosis and Treatment Can Save Your Life

GENERAL INFORMATION ABOUT MALE BREAST CANCER

Many people do not realize that men have breast tissue and that they can develop breast cancer. Men at any age may develop breast cancer, but it is usually detected in men between 60 and 70 years of age. According to the American Cancer Society, in 2005 some 1,690 new cases of invasive breast cancer were diagnosed among men in the United States. Male breast cancer makes up less than 1% of all cases of breast cancer. One in every one hundred breast cancer cases is a man.

Although the number of breast cancer incidents is far greater in women, men need to know that the disease is just as debilitating for them. The impact is the same; most times the outcome is different.

Anatomy of the Male Breasts
Until puberty, young boys and girls have a small amount of breast tissue consisting of a few ducts (tubular passages) located under the nipple and areola (area around the nipple). At puberty, a girl's ovaries produce female hormones, causing breast ducts to grow, lobules (milk glands) to form at the ends of ducts, and the amount of stroma (fatty and connective tissue surrounding ducts and lobules) to increase. On the other hand, male hormones produced by the testicles prevent further growth of breast tissue. Men's breast tissue contains ducts, but only a few if any lobules. Like all cells of the body, a man's breast duct cells can undergo cancerous changes.

Warning Signs
The most common symptom is a lump in the breast area. However, other signs may occur such as a change in the size or shape of the breast, an ulcer on the skin, fluid coming out of the nipple (discharge) or turning in of the nipple (inversion). Another possible symptom is a rash on the nipple or surrounding area.

Early Diagnosis and Treatment Can Save Your Life

Types
- **_Infiltrating ductal carcinoma_**: Cancer that has spread beyond the cells lining ducts in the breast. Most men with beast cancer have this type of cancer.
- **_Ductile carcinoma in situ_**: Abnormal cells that are found in the lining of a duct; also called intraductal carcinoma.
- **_Inflammatory breast cancer_**: A type of cancer in which the breast looks red and swollen and feels warm.
- **_Paget's disease of the nipple_**: A tumor that has grown from ducts beneath the nipple onto the surface of the nipple.

Risk Factors
- Exposure to radiation.
- Having a disease related to high levels of estrogen in the body, such as cirrhosis (liver disease) or Klinefelter's syndrome (a genetic disorder where an extra female chromosome is present).
- Having several female relatives who have had breast cancer, especially relatives who have an alteration of the BRCA2 gene.

Tests Used to Detect and Diagnose
A doctor should be seen if changes in the breasts are noticed. Typically, men with breast cancer have lumps that can be felt. Some or all of the following tests can be performed to detect breast cancer.
- Mammogram (breast x-ray): Mammograms may be used to look for changes in the breast, but ultrasound is generally more helpful for diagnosing breast cancer in men.
- Ultrasound scan: A scan using sound waves is used to see whether a lump is solid or contains fluid. A small amount of clear gel is applied to the beast area. Then a small microphone-like device is rubbed over the area to show a picture of the breast on a monitor screen.
- Needle biopsy: The removal of part of a lump, suspicious tissue, or fluid, using a thin needle. This procedure is also called a fine-needle aspiration biopsy.

Early Diagnosis and Treatment Can Save Your Life

- Core biopsy: The removal of part of a lump or suspicious tissue using a wide needle.
- **_Excisional biopsy:_** The removal of an entire lump or suspicious tissue.

Factors That Affect Prognosis (chance of recovery) and Treatment Options

The prognosis and treatment options depend on the following:
- The stage of the cancer (whether it is in the breast only or has spread to other places in the body.)
- The type of breast cancer.
- Certain characteristics of the cancer cells.
- Whether the cancer is found in the other breast.
- The patient's age and general health.

Treatment Option Overview

Different types of treatments are available for men with breast cancer. Some treatments are standard (the currently used treatment), and some are being tested in clinical trials. Before starting treatment, patients may want to think about taking part in a clinical trial. Choosing the most appropriate cancer treatment is a decision that ideally involves the patient, family, and health care team. Four types of standard treatment are used to treat men with breast cancer:

> **Surgery** for men with breast cancer is usually a modified radical mastectomy (removal of the breast, some of the lymph nodes under the arm, the lining over the chest muscles, and sometimes part of the chest wall muscles). Some of the lymph nodes under the arm may also be removed and examined under a microscope.
>
> **Chemotherapy** is a cancer treatment that uses drugs to stop the growth of cancer cells, either by killing the cells or by stopping the cells from dividing. When chemotherapy is taken by mouth or injected into a vein or muscle, the drugs enter the bloodstream and can reach cancer cells throughout the body (systemic chemotherapy). When chemotherapy is placed directly in the spinal column, a body

Early Diagnosis and Treatment Can Save Your Life

cavity such as the abdomen, or an organ, the drugs mainly affect cancer cells in those areas. The way the chemotherapy is given depends on the type and stage of the cancer being treated.

Hormone therapy is a cancer treatment that removes hormones or blocks their action and stops cancer cells from growing. Hormones are substances produced by glands in the body and circulated in the bloodstream. The presence of some hormones can cause certain can-cers to grow. If tests show that the cancer cells have places were hormones can attach (receptors), drugs, surgery, or radiation therapy are used to reduce the production of hormones or block them from working.

Radiation therapy is a cancer treatment that uses high-energy x-rays or other types of radiation to kill cancer cells. There are two types of radiation therapy. External radiation therapy uses a machine outside the body to send radiation toward the cancer. Internal radiation therapy uses a radioactive substance sealed in needles, seeds, wires, or catheters that are placed directly into or near the cancer. The way the radiation therapy is given depends on the type and stage of the cancer being treated.

Other types of treatment are being tested in clinical trials. Information about ongoing clinical trails is available from the National Cancer Institute (NCI) Website: www.cancer.gov.

Survival
Survival for men with breast cancer is similar to that for women with breast cancer when their stage at diagnosis is the same. Breast cancer in men, however, is often diagnosed at a later stage. Cancer found at a later stage maybe less likely to be cured.

The prognosis (outlook) for men with breast cancer was once thought to be worse than that for women, but this is not true. Stage for stage, the survival rates are equal. In other words, men and women with each stage of breast cancer have a similar outlook for survival.

Early Diagnosis and Treatment Can Save Your Life

16

Know Your Rights... You Have A Right To Know

Patients have both rights and responsibilities when it comes to their health and the health care services they receive. It is important that you know what they are. Many patients lose their jobs or are denied insurance coverage. Some who don't have insurance when diagnosed fall through the cracks. Often your insurance carriers or HMO will refuse to pay for a particular treatment or medicine or will cancel your coverage. Even if you are uninsured, you have rights. Know what your rights are so that you will recognize when you are not receiving fair and effective treatment. For this reason alone, knowing your rights will enable you to take a proactive role in the decisions that affect your health care and your life.

On March 26, 1997, President Bill Clinton appointed an Advisory Commission on Consumer Protection and Quality in the Health Care Industry. The Commission issued its final report, "Quality First: Better Health Care for All Americans," in March 1998. As part of its work, the Commission issued a Consumer Bill of Rights and Responsibilities. This document was intended to serve as a blueprint for how systems and procedures that aim to protect consumers and ensure quality of care could be improved. The Patient's Bill of Rights and Responsibilities expressed three major objectives:

- To strengthen consumer confidence by assuring that the health care system is fair and responsive to consumers' needs, provides consumers with credible and effective mechanisms to address their concerns, and encourages consumers to take an active role in improving and assuring their health.
- To reaffirm the importance of a strong relationship between patients and their health care professionals.
- To reaffirm the critical role consumers play in safeguarding their health by establishing rights and responsibilities for all participants in improving their health.

PATIENTS' BILL OF RIGHTS

I. **Information Disclosure**
You have the right to receive accurate and easily understood information about your health plan, health care professionals, and health care facilities. If you speak another language, have a physical or mental disability, or just don't understand something, assistance will be provided so you can make informed health care decisions.

II. **Choice of Providers and Plans**
You have the right to a choice of health care providers that is sufficient to provide you with access to appropriate high-quality health care.

Early Diagnosis and Treatment Can Save Your Life

III. Access to Emergency Services

If you have severe pain, an injury, or sudden illness that convinces you that your health is in serious jeopardy, you have the right to receive screening and stabilization emergency services whenever and wherever needed, without prior authorization or financial penalty.

IV. Participation in Treatment Decisions

You have the right to know all your treatment options and to participate in decisions about your care. Parents, guardians, family members, or other individuals that you designate can represent you if you cannot make your own decisions.

V. Respect and Nondiscrimination

You have a right to considerate, respectful, and nondiscriminatory care from your doctors, health plan representatives, and other health care providers.

VI. Confidentiality of Health Information

You have the right to talk in confidence with health care providers and to have your health care information protected. You also have the right to review and copy your own medical record and request that your physician amend your record if it is not accurate, relevant, or complete.

VII. Complaints and Appeals

You have the right to a fair, fast, and objective review of any complaint you have against your health plan, doctors, hospitals or other health care personnel. This includes complaints regarding waiting times, operating hours, the conduct of health care personnel, and the adequacy of health care facilities.

Early Diagnosis and Treatment Can Save Your Life

WOMEN'S HEALTH AND CANCER RIGHTS ACT

On October 21, 1998, the Women's Health and Cancer Rights Act (WHCRA) was signed into law. This law contains important new protections for breast cancer patients who elect breast reconstruction with a mastectomy. The Department of Labor and Department of Health and Human Services oversee it.

WHCRA requires all group health plans and health insurance issuers, including insurance companies and health maintenance organizations (HMOs), to notify women about the coverage it requires when the person enrolls for insurance and yearly thereafter. It mandates that coverage provide for mastectomy related services, including reconstruction and surgery to achieve symmetry between the breasts, prostheses, and complications resulting from a mastectomy (including lymphedema). Several states also have their own laws requiring health plans that cover mastectomies to provide coverage for reconstructive surgery after a mastectomy. However, not all health plans are subject to state law. This law covers those plans not currently covered by state law and sets a minimum standard securing this service for all women in all states. This includes those with weaker state laws and those without any laws on this at all.

Although the law went into effect on October 21, 1998, it is a somewhat complicated and complex measure. If you have questions or concern about the new law, please contact the Department of Labor's toll-free number at 800-998-7542. You can also call your health plan directly (a number should be listed on your insurance card) or your State Insurance Commissioner's office (a number should be located in your local phone book under "State Government").

Under the Women's Health Act, group health plans, insurance companies, and HMOs that offer mastectomy coverage must also pro-

Early Diagnosis and Treatment Can Save Your Life

vide coverage for reconstruction surgery after mastectomy. This coverage includes reconstruction of the breast removed by mastectomy, reconstruction of the other breast to produce a symmetrical appearance, breast prostheses, and treatment of physical complications at all stages of the mastectomy, including lymphedema.

This law sets a federal floor so that women can obtain breast reconstruction following mastectomy even if they live in states that do not require insurance companies to provide this coverage.

Early Diagnosis and Treatment Can Save Your Life

YOUR PROTECTION UNDER THE LAW

PROTECTION AGAINST JOB DIESCRIMINATION

The Americans With Disabilities Act (ADA)
The ADA bans discrimination by both private and public employers against qualified workers who have disabilities or histories of disability. Although the ADA does not specifically include cancer survivors, it is expected that survivors will be included based on past legal rulings.

As of July 26, 1994, the ADA covers private employers with fifteen or more workers. Under this law, employers:

- Cannot require you to take pre-employment exams designed to screen out people with disabilities such as a history of cancer.
- Can ask you medical questions only after you are offered employment and only if the questions relate specifically to the job.
- Cannot treat workers with disabilities differently from other workers. Their disability must not affect their pay, promotions, insurance and pension benefits, vacation time, job training, or continued employment.
- Must make a "reasonable accommodation" to allow you to do your job.
- Cannot punish an employee for filing a discrimination complaint.
- Cannot discriminate against the family members of a disabled person because of the relationship. For example, employers cannot treat your spouse differently because they assume he or she will take leave time to care for you.

Complaints filed under this law are handled by the local offices of the Equal Employment Opportunities Commission (EEOC). You can find the office nearest you by calling 800-872-3362.

Early Diagnosis and Treatment Can Save Your Life

FEDERAL REHABILITATION ACT

This law protects cancer survivors in hiring practices, promotion, transfers, and lay-offs on the federal level. Federal employees file complaints with the agency the employ them. Those who work for companies that receive money from federal agencies file complaints with the funding agency.

STATE LAWS

Most states also have laws forbidding job discrimination against people with disabilities. Many have rules similar to those of the ADA. In some states, however, cancer survivors are not protected under these laws because they only cover people with physical handicaps. To enforce your rights under state law, you must file a complaint with your state enforcement agency. To find out about the laws in your state or where to file a complaint, contact the EEOC Public Information System at 800-669-4000. You can also check in your local telephone book under "State Government."

FILING DEADLINES

If you do plan to file a legal complaint, be sure to meet the proper deadlines. Most complaints to federal and state agencies must be made within 180 days of a problem. Time periods can be shorter, however. For instance, if you are a federal employee filing under the Federal Rehabilitation Act, you have only 30 days to state your complaint.

THE RIGHT TO MEDICAL LEAVE

THE FAMILY AND MEDICAL LEAVE ACT OF 1993

This law requires employers with 50 or more employees to provide unpaid leave to employees with a serious illness or family members who need time to care for a seriously ill child, spouse, parent, healthy newborn or newly adopted child. Some of its specifics benefits include:

- Allows up to 12 weeks of unpaid leave during any 12-month period.
- Requires employers to continue providing health insurance and other benefits during the leave period.

Early Diagnosis and Treatment Can Save Your Life

- Requires employers to give employees the same job, or an equivalent job, when they return from leave.
- Allows employees to reduce their work schedule or work on-and-off when it is medically necessary.

Employees must make every effort to avoid disrupting the work schedule, and employers are allowed to verify a medical need. To qualify for leave under this law, an employee must have worked at least 25 hours per week for one year; companies are allowed to deny unpaid leave to their highest paid employees.

To enforce your Family Medical Leave rights, you must file a lawsuit against your employer within two years of the problem.

TO ENFORCE YOUR RIGHTS

It's usually best to try to solve problems informally with employers and insurers. If you need to further enforce your legal rights the following contact information may be useful.

- COBRA rights are enforced by:
  Pension and Welfare Benefits Administration
  U.S. Department of Labor
  200 Constitution Avenue, N.W.
  Room N-5658
  Washington, D.C. 20210

- ERISA rights are enforced by:
  Employee Benefits Security Administration
  U.S. Department of Labor
  200 Constitution Avenue, N.W.
  Room N-5658
  Washington, D.C. 20210
  202-219-8776

Early Diagnosis and Treatment Can Save Your Life

- To verify the accuracy of information on file about your health, contact:
  The Medical Information Bureau (MIB)
  P. O. Box 105 – Essex Station
  Boston, MA 02112
  617-426-3660

Ask for a form requesting disclosure of any information in your file. (You may be on file with the Bureau and not know it; the Bureau keeps files on nearly 15 million Americans for insurance companies they represent.) After your request, the MIB will send your file to your doctor, and he or she can check whether it is correct. This step is important because the information in your file may affect insurance company decisions.

Additional reading that you will find extremely helpful can be found in the pamphlet *What Cancer Survivors Need To Know About Health Insurance.* This document discusses types of insurance available, how to buy insurance, how to submit claims, and how to handle claim rejection. Available free of charge. Contact:

- National Coalition for Cancer Survivorship (NCCS)
  1010 Wayne Avenue, 7th Floor
  Silver Springs, MD 20910
  301-650-8860

Many people need help paying for medical costs that aren't covered by their insurance. For financial assistance, you may want to contact:

- Local cancer support organizations, which may provide referrals to community sources for financial aid.
- Your local office on aging if you are an older adult.
- The county board of assistance or welfare office.
- Nonprofit consumer credit counseling services in your area. If you cannot find one in the phone book, the National Foundation for Consumer Credit, Inc. (301-589-5600) can direct you to a service in your area.

Early Diagnosis and Treatment Can Save Your Life

U.S. Government

The U.S. Government has a number of programs designed to help people with low incomes or disabilities pay their bills. For information, call your local office of:

- Aid to Families With Dependent Children (AFDC) and Food Stamps programs. Look for the numbers under the local government, social services section of your telephone book.
- Medicare/Medicaid Information. Call your local Social Security office to receive an explanation of the medical costs covered. Note: For people less than age 65, Medicare coverage does not begin until two years from the date they are declared disabled.
- Social Security Administration. Call 800-772-1213 for general infor-mation on Social Security benefits you may be eligible to receive.
- The Department of Veterans Affairs. Request information about med-ical benefits for veterans and their dependents.
- The Cancer Information Services. Call 800-4-CANCER to request information about drug companies with assistance programs for cancer patients with low incomes.

Your Hospital

To find out about setting up monthly payment plans for hospital bills, contact your:

- Hospital patient advocate
- Hospital financial aid counselor
- Hospital social worker
- Patient representative in the hospital business office

Early Diagnosis and Treatment Can Save Your Life

OPTIONS FOR GETTING LIFE INSURANCE AFTER CANCER TREATMENT

Making Sense of Health Insurance:

Cancer survivors may need information and new skills to handle insurance matters. Every state (plus Puerto Rico, the Virgin Islands, and the District of Columbia) has a health insurance information and counseling services that can help. The services give you free information and help on Medicare, Medicaid, Medigap, long-term care, and other health insurance benefits. State health insurance offices provide printed information, help with choosing health insurance coverage, and even help understanding your bills, insurance claims, and explanation forms. If you have trouble reaching the office in your state using the telephone numbers listed below (the 800 numbers work only within the state), call the Medicare hotline at 800-633-4227.

Many larger companies carefully grade insurance risks by the type and stage of cancer. Depending on your diagnosis, you may be eligible for a policy. Before choosing and insurance carrier, consider the following:

- Get prices from several companies. Policy costs can vary a great deal among companies.
- Request group insurance through a professional, fraternal, membership, or political organization to which you belong.
- Consider a policy with limited benefits (a "graded" policy) if you cannot get full death benefits.

The following directory provides phone numbers for State Health Insurance Counseling and Information Offices and Peer Review Organizations (PROs). PROs are groups of practicing doctors and other health care professionals paid by the federal government to monitor the quality of care provided to Medicare patients by hospitals, skilled care facilities, home health agencies, managed care plans, and ambulatory surgical centers.

Early Diagnosis and Treatment Can Save Your Life

State	Counseling and Information Office/Local No.	PeerReview Organization
Alabama	800-243-5463 (334-242-5743)	800-760-3540
Alaska	800-478-6065 (907-269-3680)	800-445-6941
American Samoa	808-586-7299 (888-875-9229)	800-524-6550
Arizona	800-432-4040 (602-542-6595)	800-626-1577
Arkansas	800-224-6330 (501-371-2782)	800-272-5528
California	800-434-0222 (916-323-6525)	800-841-1602
Colorado	800-544-9181 (303-899-7499)	800-727-7086
Connecticut	800-994-9422 (860-424-5245)	800-553-7590
Delaware	800-336-9500 (302-739-6266)	800-642-8686
District of Columbia	202-676-3900 (202-739-0668)	DC: 800-999-3362 MD: 800-492-5811
Florida	800-963-5337 (850-414-2060)	800-844-0795
Georgia	800-669-8387 (404-657-5334)	800-982-0411
Guam	888-875-9229 (808-586-7299)	800-524-6550
Hawaii	808-586-7299	800-524-6550 Oahu: 808-545-2550
Idaho	800-247-4422 (208-334-4350)	800-445-6941
Illinois	800-548-9034 (217-782-0004)	800-647-8089
Indiana	800-452-4800 (317-233-3475)	800-288-1499
Iowa	800-351-4664 (515-281-6867)	800-752-7014
Kansas	800-860-5260 (316-337-7386)	800-432-0407
Kentucky	877-293-7447 (502-564-7372)	800-288-1499
Louisiana	800-259-5301 (225-342-5301)	800-433-4958
Maine	800-262-2232 (207-287-9200)	800-722-0151
Maryland	800-243-3425 (410-767-1100)	800-492-5811
Massachusetts	800-882-2003 (617-727-7750)	800-252-5533
Michigan	800-803-7174 (517-886-0899)	800-365-5899
Minnesota	800-333-2433	800-444-3423

Early Diagnosis and Treatment Can Save Your Life

State	Counseling and Information Office/Local No.		PeerReview Organization
Mississippi	800-948-3090	(601-359-4929)	800-844-0600
Missouri	800-390-3330		800-347-1016
Montana	800-332-2272	(406-444-7781)	800-497-8232
Nebraska	800-234-7119	(402-471-2201)	800-247-3004
Nevada	800-307-4444	(702-486-3478)	800-748-6773
New Hampshire	800-852-3388	(603-225-9000)	800-772-0151
New Jersey	800-792-8820	(609-588-3139)	800-624-4557
New Mexico	800-432-2080	(505-827-7640)	800-279-6824
New York	800-333-4114		800-331-7767
North Carolina	800-443-9354	(919-733-01110)	800-722-0468
North Dakota	800-247-0560	(701-328-2440)	800-472-2902
Ohio	800-686-1578	(614-644-3458)	800-589-7337
Oklahoma	800-763-2828	(405-521-6628)	800-522-3414
Oregon	800-722-4134	(503-947-7263)	800-344-4354
Pennsylvania	800-783-7067	(717-783-8975)	800-222-0711
Puerto Rico	800-981-4355	(787-721-8590)	787-753-6705
Rhode Island	401-462-3000	(401-462-0508)	800-553-7590
South Carolina	800-868-9095	(803-898-2850)	800-633-4227
South Dakota	800-822-8804	(605-733-3656)	800-658-2285
Tennessee	877-801-0044		800-489-4633
Texas	800-252-9240	(512-424-6840)	800-725-8315
Utah	800-541-7735	(801-538-3910)	800-274-2290
Vermont	800-642-5119	(802-865-0360)	800-772-0151
Virgin Islands	809-778-6311		809-778-6470
Virginia	800-552-3402	(804-662-9333)	800-545-3814
Washington	800-397-4422	(206-654-1833)	800-445-6941
West Virginia	800-642-9004	(304-558-3317)	800-642-8686
Wisconsin	800-242-1060	(608-267-3201)	800-362-2320
Wyoming	800-856-4398	(307-856-6880)	800-497-8232

Early Diagnosis and Treatment Can Save Your Life

17

Where To Go, Who To Call

Depending on where you live, there are a number of support groups and local community organizations, including churches that are available to help you. The American Cancer Society has a local presence in all the states. Your local health department is also a good place to start. If there's no organization in your community at the local level, there are a number of national organizations that are very knowledgeable and extremely helpful. Some of these agencies provide everything from advocacy and networking to legal rights information, referral services, outreach, support groups, and educational tools. Some of these services are available to breast cancer survivors as well as family members of survivors or for those who care for them. Don't hesitate to call any one or all of them if you need help.

NATIONAL BREAST CANCER ORGANIZATIONS

African American Breast Cancer Alliance (AABCA) P.O. Box 8981, Minneapolis, MN 55408, 612-825-3675. A member supported advocacy and support group dedicated to providing hope, awareness, education, emotional and social support to breast cancer survivors, their family members and the community. Email: aabcainc@yahoo.com. Web site: www.aabcainc.org.

American Cancer Society (ACS) has voluntary programs concerned with breast cancer in its divisions and units nationwide, as well as national programs in research and advocacy. The ACS tollfree hot line, 800-ACS-2345, provides information on all forms of cancer and refer rals to the ACS sponsored "Reach to Recovery" and "Look Good, Feel Better" programs. For more information, contact your local American Cancer Society office or visit their Web site: www.cancer.org.

American Society of Plastic Surgeons (ASPS) The mission of the ASPS is to advance quality care to plastic surgery patients by encouraging high standards of training, ethics, physician practice and research in plastic surgery. The society advocates for patient safety, such as requiring its members to operate in accredited surgical facilities that have passed rigorous external review of equipment and staffing. 444 East Algonquin Road, Arlington Heights, IL 60005. Plastic Surgeon Referral Service: 888-475-2784. Web site: www.plasticsurgery.org.

Avon's Breast Cancer Awareness Crusade The goal of the Avon Foundation Breast Cancer Crusade is to benefit all women through research, clinical care, education and support services. There is special emphasis on reaching medically underserved women, including low-income, elderly and minority women, and women without adequate health insurance. Web site: www.avoncompany.com.

Early Diagnosis and Treatment Can Save Your Life

Black Women For Wellness A resource center for black women, working at the crossroads of black poverty and wealth, connecting women with each other for enhanced health and well being. For more information call: 323-290-5955. Or write: 3460 Wilshire Blvd., Suite 1102, Los Angeles, CA. Web site: www.bwwla.com.

Black Women's Health Imperative (New name for National Black Women's Health Project.) Seeks to develop and communicate highly effective and beneficial health information, products and programs to African American women. Offer the tools and information for women to give themselves the best self-care to prevent health problems before they occur, to recognize symptoms and early warning signs and to understand all of the options available for their specific health situations. Can be contacted at: 600 Pennsylvania Ave., SE, Ste. 310, Washington, D.C. 20003, 202-548-4000.

Breast Cancer Fund provides funding for advocacy, support, education as well as research into better ways to prevent, detect, and treat breast cancer. Founded in 1992, the Breast Cancer Fund works from the knowledge that breast cancer is not simply a personal tragedy, but a public health priority that demands action from all.1388 Sutter Street, Ste. 400, San Francisco, Ca. 94109-5400, 415-346-8223.Web site: www.breastcancerfund.org. E-mail: info@breastcancerfund.org.

Breast Cancer Resource Committee is dedicated to reducing the incidence and mortality of cancer among African American women, particularly those women who have little or no access to adequate health care and treatment. Founded in 1989 by Zora Kramer-Brown, BCRC is a response to the immense need in the African American community for increased education and understanding about breast cancer risk factors, the importance of breast cancer screening and early detection, and the availability of successful treatment options and support. 2005 Belmont Street, NW, Washington, DC 20009, 202-463-8040. Web site: www.bcresource.org.

Early Diagnosis and Treatment Can Save Your Life

Canadian Cancer Society (National Office) A national community-based organization of volunteers whose mission is the eradication of cancer and the enhancement of the quality of life of people living with cancer. Suite 200, 10 Alcorn Avenue, Toronto, Ontario M4V 3B1. Phone: 416-961-7223. General e-mail: ccs@cancer.ca.

Cancer Care, Inc. A national non-profit organization that provides professional support services to anyone affected by cancer: people with cancer, caregivers, children, loved ones, and the bereaved. Cancer Care programs, including counseling, education, financial assistance and practical help, are provided by trained oncology social workers and are completely free of charge. National office is located at 275 Seventh Avenue, New York, NY 10001, 212-712-8400. Toll free: 800- 813-HOPE (800-813-4673). Web site: www.cancercare.org. Email: info@cancercare.org.

Cancer Information Service of the National Cancer Institute, a national information and education network, is a free public service of the NCI, the federal government's primary agency for cancer research. The CIS meets the information needs of patients, the public, and health professionals. Specially trained staff provide the latest scientific information in understandable language. CIS staff answer questions in English and Spanish and distributes NCI materials. Call 800-4 CANCER (800-422-6237). TTY: 800-332-8615.Web site: wwwicic.nci.nih.gov.

Celebrating Life is one of the leading foundations in the nation that is dedicated to educating the African American community and women of color about the risks of breast cancer, to encouraging advancements in the early detection and treatment, and to improving survival rates among these women. Can be contacted at P. O. Box 224076, Dallas, TX 75222-4076 or call 800-207-0992. Web site: www.celebratinglife.org.

Gilda's Club Worldwide. Through workshops, social activities and network groups, Gilda's Club provides crucial emotional support. There are currently 13 U.S. offices, open to anyone affected by cancer, and all serv-

Early Diagnosis and Treatment Can Save Your Life

ices are free. Gilda's Club is named for Gilda Radner, the comedian who died of ovarian cancer in 1989. Its mission: To approach the disease with a positive spirit similar to hers. Can be reached at 888-GILDA-4-U. By mail at 332 Eighth Ave., Suite 1402, New York, NY 10001. Web site: www.gildasclub.org.

Susan G. Komen Breast Cancer Foundation is a national organization with a network of volunteers working through local chapters and Race for the Cure events across the country funding education and screening projects in local communities for the medically underserved. Their mission is to eradicate breast cancer as a life- threatening disease by advancing research, education, screening and treatment. The Komen Foundation remains the nation's largest private funder of research dedicated solely to breast cancer. For information about breast health or breast cancer call 800-I'M AWARE (800-462-9273). Web site: www.komen.org.

National Breast Cancer Coalition (NBCC) is a grassroots advocacy organization committed to the eradication of the breast cancer epidemic. The NBCC's goals are: To increase the money available for research into breast cancer and to focus research on finding the cause and cure for this insidious disease; to make certain that all women have access to the quality breast cancer care and treatment they need, regardless of their economic circumstances; and to increase the influence of women with breast cancer in the decision making process that affects their lives. For more information, contact NBCC at 1101 17th Street, NW, Suite 1300, Washington, DC 20036, 800-622-2838. Web site: www.natlbcc.org.

National Breast and Cervical Cancer Early Detection Program. Helps low-income, uninsured, and underserved women gain access to lifesaving early detection screening programs for breast and cervical cancers. For general cancer information contact CDC's cancer prevention and control at: Division of Cancer Prevention and Control, National Center for Chronic Disease Prevention and Health Promotion, Centers for Disease Control and Prevention, 4770 Buford Highway, NE, MS K-64, Atlanta, GA. 30341-3717. Call: 888-842-6355. Web site: www.cdc.gov.

Early Diagnosis and Treatment Can Save Your Life

National Cancer Institute (NCI) - U.S. National Institutes of Health. The National Cancer Institute coordinates the National Cancer Program, which conducts and supports research, training, health information dissemination, and other programs with respect to the cause, diagnosis, prevention, and treatment of cancer, rehabilitation from cancer, and the continuing care of cancer patients and the families of cancer patients. NCI's central Web site (www.cancer.gov) has extensive information on cancer prevention, treatment, statistics, research, clinical trials, and news. Information specialists from the NCI's Cancer Information Services can be reached at: 800-4-CANCER 800-422-6237.

National Coalition for Cancer Survivorship. (NCCS) raises awareness of cancer survivorship through its publications, quarterly newsletter, and education to eliminate the stigma of cancer, and advocacy for insurance, employment, and legal rights for people with cancer. NCCS also facilitates networking among cancer programs, serves as an information clearinghouse, and encourages the study of cancer survivorship. On a national level, NCCS provides public policy leadership on legislative, regulatory and financing matters and promotes responsible advocacy among national cancer organizations. For more information, contact NCCS at 1010 Wayne Avenue, Suite 770, Silver Spring, MD 20910, 301-650-9127. Web site: www.canceradvocacy.org. E-mail address: info@canceradvocacy.org

National Lymphedema Network (NLN). Its mission is to create awareness of lymphedema through education and to promote and support the availability of quality medical treatment for all individuals at risk for or affected by lymphedema. Address: Latham Square, 1611 Telegraph Ave., Suite 1111, Oakland, CA 94612-2138. Call: 800-541-3259 or 510-208-3200.

National Women's Health Information Center (NWHIC). The National Women's Health Information Center, sponsored by the U.S. Public Health Service's Office on Women's Health and the Department of Defense, provides a centralized point of access to women's health information from the federal government and the private sector. To obtain information on breast cancer and other topics, call the NWHIC's toll free number, 800-994-9662. Web site: www.4woman.gov.

Early Diagnosis and Treatment Can Save Your Life

John W. Nick Foundation, Inc. Was originally established November 1995 to promote awareness of male breast cancer. Since its inception, research has shown that male breast cancer is a bigger problem that people realized, due in part to the fact that men are misdiagnosed or ashamed to come forward about their disease. Web site: www.johnwnickfoundation.org. Call: 772-589-1440.

SHARE. This organization offers peer-led support groups in English and Spanish (with a capacity in 12 other languages) to women with breast or ovarian cancer and their families and friends. Located in New York City, SHARE provides survivor-led support groups, wellness programs, educational forums and outreach and advocacy activities. Its hotlines are answered 24 hours a day and are staffed by multilingual volunteers who will help you find resources wherever you live. Mailing address: 1501 Broadway, Suite 704A, New York, NY 10036. Phone numbers are 212-719-0364; toll free: 886-891-2392. You can also contact SHARE at its website at www.share-cancersupport.org.

Sisters Network, Inc. (SNI). Founded in 1994, SNI is the first national African American breast cancer survivorship organization. Its outreach initiatives continue to promote the importance of breast health through personal empowerment, support, breast education programs, resources, information, and research through its strong affiliate chapter base. National Headquarters: 8787 Woodway Drive, Ste. 4206, Houston, TX 77063 or call 713-781-0255. Toll free: 866-781-8998. Website:www.sisternetwork-inc.org. E-mail: infonet@sistersnetworkinc.org.

The Wellness Community (TWC) is an international non-profit organization dedicated to providing support, education and hope for all people affected by cancer – at no cost. There are 22 Wellness Communities across the United States. National Headquarters: 919 18th Street, NW, Ste. 54, Washington, DC 20006. Toll free: 888-793-WELL or 202-659-9709.

Early Diagnosis and Treatment Can Save Your Life

Women's Information Network Against Breast Cancer – A nonprofit organization dedicated to increasing public awareness about breast cancer and ensuring that individuals from all cultural and socioeconomic backgrounds receive equal and rapid access to quality health care based on evidence-based treatment guidelines and state-of-the-art support, education and information about the disease. Contact by mail at: WIN Against Breast Cancer, 536 S. Second Ave., Suite K, Covina, CA 91723-3043. Contact toll free (U.S. only) at: 866-294-6222; phone: 626-332-2255. Web site: www.winabc.org. E-mail: mail@winabc.org.

Young Survival Coalition (YSC) is the only international non-profit network of breast cancer survivors and supporters dedicated to the issues and concerns unique to young women with breast cancer. Through action, advocacy and awareness, the YSC seeks to educate the medical, research, breast cancer and legislative communities and persuade them to address breast cancer in women 40 and under. The Young Survival Coalition also serves as a point of contact for young women living with breast cancer. Mailing address: Young Survival Coalition, 155 6th Avenue, 10th Floor, New York, NY 10013. Phone: 212-206-6610. Web site: www.youngsurvival.org.

Y-ME National Breast Cancer Organization provides breast cancer-information, support and referrals through their national, 24 hour, toll-free hot line, 800-221-2141; Spanish services available, 800-986-9505. The mission of Y-ME National Breast Cancer Organization is to ensure, through information, empowerment and peer support, that no one faces breast cancer alone. YME has also started a hot line for men whose partners have had breast cancer. Call or write to 212 W. Van Buren Street, Ste. 1000, Chicago, IL , 60607-3903. Phone: 312-986-8338. Web site: www.yme.org.

Early Diagnosis and Treatment Can Save Your Life

The YWCA of the U.S.A.'s Encore Plus Program located in member associations throughout the U.S.A., provides early detection outreach, education, postdiagnostic support and exercise to all women. To find the location of the program nearest to you, call 800-872-9622.

Early Diagnosis and Treatment Can Save Your Life

Chartered Divisions of the American Cancer Society, Inc.

California Division, Inc.
1710 Webster Street
Oakland, CA 94612
510-893-7900 - office
510-835-8656 - fax

Great West Division, Inc.
(AK, AZ, CO, ID, MT, ND,
NM, NV, OR, UT, WA, WY)
2120 First Avenue North
Seattle, WA 98100-1140
206-283-1152 - office
206-285-3469 - fax

Eastern Division, Inc.
(LI, NJ, NYC, NYS, Queens,
and Westchester)
6725 Lyons Street
East Syracuse, NY 13057
315-437-7025 - office
315-437-0540 - fax

Heartland Division, Inc.
(KS, MO, NE, OK)
1100 Pennsylvania Avenue
Kansas City, MO 64105
816-842-7111 - office
816-842-8828 - fax

Florida Division, Inc.
(includ. Puerto Rico Operations)
3709 West Jetton Avenue
Tampa, FL 33629-5146
813-253-0541 - office
813-254-5857 - fax

Illinois Division, Inc.
225 N. Michigan Ave. Ste. 1200
Chicago, IL 60601
312-641-6150 - office
312-641-3533 - fax

Puerto Rico
Calle Alverio #577
Esquina Sargento Medina
Hata Rey, PR 00918
787-764-2295 - office
787-764-0553 - fax

Mid-South Division, Inc.
(AL, AR, KY, LA, MS, TN)
1100 Ireland Way, Suite 300
Birmingham, AL 35205-7014
205-930-8860 - office
205-930-8877 - fax

Early Diagnosis and Treatment Can Save Your Life

Where To Go, Who To Call

Great Lakes Division, Inc.
(MI, IN)
1755 Abbey Road
East Lansing, MI 48823-1907
517-332-2222 - office
517-664-1498 - fax

New England Division, Inc.
(CT, ME, MA, NH, RI, VT)
30 Speen Street
Framingham, MA 01701-9376
508-270-4600 - office
508-270-4699 - fax

Ohio Division, Inc.
5555 Frantz Road
Dublin, OH 43017
614-889-9565 - office
614-889-6578 - fax

Pennsylvania Division, Inc.
(PA, Phil)
Route 422 and Sipe Avenue
Hershey, PA 17033-0897
717-533-6144 - office
717-534-1075 - fax

Midwest Division, Inc.
(IA, MN, SD, WI)
8364 Hickman Road, Suite D
Des Moines, IA 50325
515-253-0147 - office
515-253-0806 - fax

South Atlantic Division
(DC, DE, GA, MD, NC, SC, VA, WV)
2200 Lake Boulevard
Atlanta, GA 30319
404-816-7800 - office
404-816-9443 - fax

Texas Division, Inc.
(including Hawaii Pacific opertions)
2433 Ridgepoint Drive
Austin, TX 78754
512-919-1800 - office
512-919-1844 - fax

Hawaii Pacific, Inc.
2370 Nuuanu Avenue
Honolulu, HI 96817
808-595-7500 - office
808-595-7502 - fax

Early Diagnosis and Treatment Can Save Your Life

18

Words You Need To Know

This section contains words and phrases that will help you in the event that you or someone you love are ever diagnosed with this life altering disease. You don't have to memorize them, but become familiar with them so you can communicate with your doctor without feeling so overwhelmed. Knowing how to effectively convey your concerns and understanding your doctor's responses to your questions alleviates some of the stress associated with any illness.

Early Diagnosis and Treatment Can Save Your Life

a

ablative therapy. To surgically remove a body part or to destroy its function (for example, some forms of chemotherapy ablate the ovaries, thus causing infertily).

abscess. A pocket of pus that forms as the body's defenses attempt to wall off infection-causing germs.

acini. The sac-like part of the milk-producing glands in the breast. These are also called lobules.

adenocarcinoma. Cancer that starts in the glands, such as in the lobules of the breast.

adenoma. A benign growth that may or may not transform to cancer (see also fibroadenoma).

adjuvant (ad-joo'-vant) therapy. Treatment that is added to increase the effectiveness of a primary therapy. It usually refers to chemotherapy or radiation added after surgery to kill any cancer cells still remaining and to increase the chances of curing the disease or keeping it in check.

adrenal gland. A gland near the kidney. It produces adrenaline, cortisone (in very small amounts), androgen (the "male" hormone), progestin, and possibly estrogen (the "female" hormone; most estrogen is produced in the ovaries).

advanced cancer. A stage of cancer in which the disease has spread from the primary site to other parts of the body, directly or by traveling through the network of lymph glands (lymphatics) or in the bloodstream. When the cancer has spread only to the surrounding areas, it is called locally advanced.

Early Diagnosis and Treatment Can Save Your Life

alopecia (al"o-pe'she-ah). Hair loss. This often occurs as a result of chemotherapy or radiation therapy to the head.

alternative treatment. See **therapy.**

androgen. A male sex hormone, such as testosterone. Androgens may be used to treat recurrence of breast cancer. Their effect is to block the activity of estrogen, which "feeds" some cancers.

anesthesia. The loss of feeling or sensation as a result of drugs or gases. General anesthesia causes loss of consciousness ("puts you to sleep"). Local anesthesia numbs only a specified area.

aneuploid (an'-u-ploid). Most cancer cells are aneuploid which means there is an abnormal amount of DNA in them.

antibiotic. The word means "destructive of life." Antibiotics are chemical substances, produced by living organisms or synthesized (created) in laboratories, for the purpose of killing other organisms that cause disease. Some cancer therapies interfere with the body's ability to fight off infection (they suppress the immune system), so antibiotics may be needed along with the cancer treatment to protect against or kill infectious diseases.

antibody. A protein in the blood that defends against invading foreign agents, such as a virus. The invading agent is called an antigen. Each antibody works against a specific antigen. See also **antigen.**

antiestrogen (an"te-es'tro-gen). Any substance (for example, the drug Tamoxifen) that blocks the effects of estrogen on tumors. Anti-estrogens are used to treat breast cancers that depend on estrogen for growth.

antigen (an'-ti-jen). An invading foreign agent, such as a virus, that causes antibodies to form. See also **antibodies.**

Early Diagnosis and Treatment Can Save Your Life

antimetabolites (an"ti-me-tab'o-lites). Antimetabolites are substances that interfere with the body's metabolic processes, such as burning calories or division of cells to form new cells. In treating cancer, antimetabolite drugs disrupt DNA production, which in turn prevents cell division and growth of tumors. See also **DNA**.

areola (ah-re'o-lah). The dark area of flesh that encircles the nipple of the breast.

aromatase inhibitors. Drugs that block production of estrogens by the adrenal gland. They are used to treat hormone-sensitive breast cancer in post-menopausal women. These include anastrozole, letrozole, and exemestane.

aspirate (as'pi-rat'). Removal of fluid or cells from a breast lump. See also **needle aspiration**.

asymptomatic. To be without noticeable signs or symptoms of disease. Many cancers can develop and grow without producing symptoms, especially in the early stages. Detection tests, such as mammography, try to discover developing cancers at the asymptomatic stage, when the chances for cure are usually highest. See also **screening.**

atypical. Not usual; abnormal. Cancer is the result of atypical cell division.

axilla. The armpit.

axillary node dissection. A surgical procedure in which the lymph nodes in the armpit (axillary nodes) are removed and examined, to find if breast cancer has spread to those nodes.

Early Diagnosis and Treatment Can Save Your Life

b

benign (be-nin'). Not cancer; not malignant. The main types of benign breast problems are fibroadenomas, fibrocystic changes, and cysts.

bilateral. Affecting both sides of the body; for example, bilateral breast cancer is cancer occurring in both breasts at the same time (synchronous) or at different times (metachronous).

biopsy (bi'op-se). A procedure in which tissue samples are removed from the body for examination of their appearance under a microscope to find out if cancer or other abnormal cells are present. The biopsy can be done with a needle or by surgery.

bone marrow transplant. A complex treatment that may be used when breast cancer is advanced or has recurred. The bone marrow transplant, which was first proved successful in treating leukemia, makes it possible to use exceedingly high doses of chemotherapy that would otherwise be impossible. *Autologuous bone marrow transplant* means that the patient's own bone marrow is used. When this is not possible, it becomes necessary to find a donor whose biological characteristics (such as blood type) match or closely match the patient's. A portion of the patient's or donor's bone marrow is withdrawn, cleansed, treated, and stored. The patient is then given high doses of chemotherapy that kill the cancer cells but also destroy the remaining bone marrow, thus robbing the body of its natural ability to fight infection. The cleansed and stored marrow is given by transfusion (transplanted) to rescue the patient's immune defenses. Although it has given good results in many people, it is not yet scientifically proven to be more effective than conventional therapies in treating breast cancer. It is a risky procedure that involves a lengthy and expensive hospitalization that may not be covered by the patient's health insurance. The best place to have a bone marrow transplant is in a clinical trial at a comprehensive cancer center or other facility that has the technical skill and experience to perform it safely.

Early Diagnosis and Treatment Can Save Your Life

brain scan. An imaging method used to find abnormalities in the brain, including brain cancer and cancer that has spread to the brain from other places in the body. This procedure can be done in an outpatient clinic. It is painless, except for the needle stick when a radioactive dye is injected into a vein. The images taken will show the path of the dye and place where it accumulates, indicating an abnormality.

BRCA1. A gene located on the short arm of chromosome 17. When this gene is damaged (mutated), it places a woman at greater risk of developing breast and/or ovarian cancer, compared with women who do not have the mutation. In a woman with a BRCA1 mutation, the risk of developing breast cancer by age 50 is 50%, compared with 2% in the general population. People who have this mutated gene has a 50% chance of passing on the gene to each of their children.

breast cancer. Breast cancer is a group of related diseases in which cells within the breast become abnormal and divide without control or order, invading and damaging other tissues and organs. When cancer cells break away from the original tumor and enter the bloodstream or lymphatic system, breast cancer may spread and form secondary tumors (metastases) in other parts of the body, including vital organs. The most common types of breast cancer arise in the lining of the milk ducts or in the milkproducing glands.

How rapidly it grows, whether it will spread (metastasize) or not, and what the outcome will be varies, depending on many factors, including the type of cancer, where it begins, how soon it was detected, whether it is estrogen-receptor positive or negative, and whether it responds to the type of treatment chosen. Some of the factors that contribute to the course of breast cancer are still unknown, but one area that is under study is the effect of diet. The main types of breast cancer are **ductal carcinoma** *in situ*, **infiltrating ductal carcinoma, lobular carcinoma** *in situ*, **medullary carcinoma, and Paget's disease of the nipple**. See definitions under these headings, and also see **estrogen receptor, progesterone receptor.**

Early Diagnosis and Treatment Can Save Your Life

breast conservation therapy. Surgery to remove a breast cancer and a small amount of tissue around the cancer, without removing any other part of the breast. The procedure is also called **lumpectomy, segmental excision, limited breast surgery**, or **tylectomy**. The method may require an axillary dissection and/or radiation therapy in addition to the breast conservation surgery. See also **lumpectomy**.

breast implant. A manufactured sac that is filled with silicone gel (a synthetic material containing silicon) or saline (sterile saltwater). The sac is surgically inserted to increase breast size or restore the appearance of a breast after mastectomy.

breast reconstruction. Surgery that rebuilds the breast contour after mastectomy. A breast implant or the woman's own tissue provides the contour. If desired, the nipple and areola may also be re-created. Reconstruction can be done at the time of mastectomy or any time later. See also **mammaplasty.**

breast self-exam (BSE). A technique of checking one's own breasts for lumps or suspicious changes. The method is recommended for all women over age 20, to be done once a month, usually at a time other than the days before, during, or immediately after her menstrual period.

breast specialist. A term describing health professionals who have a dedicated interest in breast health. While they may acquire specialized knowledge in this area, medical schools and licensing boards do not teach or certify a specialty in breast care.

C

calcifications. Small deposits of calcium in tissue, which are visible on mammograms.

cancer. A general term for more than 100 diseases in which abnormal or malignant cells develop. Some exist quietly within the body for years

Early Diagnosis and Treatment Can Save Your Life

without causing a problem (this happens frequently with prostate cancer). Others are aggressive, rapidly forming tumors that may invade and destroy surrounding tissue. If cancer spreads, it usually travels through the lymph system or bloodstream to distant areas of the body.

cancer care team. The group of health professionals who cooperate in the diagnosis, planning, treatment, after care, and counseling of people with cancer. The team may include any or all of the following and others: primary care physician and/or gynecologist, nurse, pathologist, oncology specialists (medical oncologist, radiation oncologist, and hematologist), surgeon, oncology nurse specialist, oncology social worker.

cancer cell. A cell that divides and reproduces abnormally and can spread throughout the body. See also **metastasis**.

carcinogen (kar"-sin'o-jen). Any substance that causes cancer or helps cancer grow.

carcinoma (kar"-si-no'-mah). A malignant tumor that begins in the lining cells of organs. Carcinomas can occur in almost any part of the body. At least 80% of all cancers are carcinomas, and almost all breast cancers are carcinomas.

case manager. The member of a cancer care team , usually a nurse or oncology nurse specialists, who "references" by coordinating all of the patient's care and needs throughout diagnosis, treatment, and recovery.

catheter (kath-i-ter). A flexible tube used to deliver fluids into or withdraw fluids from the body.

cell. The basic unit of which all living things are made. Cells carry out basic life processes. Organs are clusters of cells that have developed specialized tasks. Cells replace themselves by splitting and forming new cells (mitosis), and it is this process that is disrupted in cancer.

Early Diagnosis and Treatment Can Save Your Life

chemotherapy. Treatment with drugs to destroy cancer cells. Chemotherapy is often used in addition to surgery or radiation or to treat cancer that has come back (recurred). See also **adjuvant therapy**.

chest wall. The muscles, bones, and joints that make up the area of the body between the neck and the abdomen.

clinical trials. Research studies with groups of patients to test new drugs or procedures or to compare standard treatments, medications and procedures with others that may be equal or better.

core biopsy. A biopsy that uses a small cutting needle to remove a sample of tissue from a breast lump.

cyclic breast changes. Normal tissue changes that occur in response to the changing levels of female hormones during the menstrual cycle. Cyclic breast changes can produce swelling, tenderness, and pain.

cyst. A fluid-filled mass that is usually harmless (benign). The fluid can be removed for analysis. See **aspiration, needle aspiration.**

cytology (si-tol'-o-je). The study or examination of cells; their origin, structure, function and pathology to determine whether they are cancerous or benign.

cytotoxic (si"-to-tok'-sik). Toxic to cells; cell-killing.

d

detection. Finding disease. Early detection means that the disease is found at an early stage, before it has grown large or spread to other sites.

diagnosis. Identifying a disease by its signs, symptoms, and laboratory findings. The earlier a diagnosis of cancer is made, the better the chance for long-term survival.

Early Diagnosis and Treatment Can Save Your Life

dimpling. A pucker or indentation of the skin; on the breast, it may be a sign of cancer.

discharge. Any fluid coming from the nipple. It may be clear, milky, bloody, gray, or green.

dissection. Surgical operation which cuts and separates tissues. In treating breast cancer, the word usually refers to removal of the axillary lymph nodes and vessels.

DNA. Abbreviation for *deoxyribonucleic acid*. One of two acids (the other is RNA) found in the nucleus of all cells. DNA holds genetic information on cell growth, division, and function.

doubling time. The time it takes for a cell to divide and double itself. The doubling time of breast cancer cells depends on many things, such as the type of tumor, the resistance of the individual's body, and the location in which it tries to grow. A single cell needs 30 doublings to reach noticeable size (1 cm)—a billion cells. Cancers vary in doubling time from 8 to 600 days, averaging 100 to 120 days. Thus, a cancer may be present for many years before it can be felt. See also **cell**.

duct. A pathway. In the breast, a passage through which milk passes from the lobule (which makes the milk) to the nipple.

ductal carcinoma *in situ*. Cancer cells that started in the milk passages (ducts) and have not penetrated the duct walls into the surrounding tissue. This is a highly curable form of breast cancer that is treated with surgery or surgery plus radiation therapy.

duct ectasia. Widening of the ducts of the breast, often related to a breast inflammation called periductal mastitis. Duct ectasia is a benign condition. Symptoms of this condition are a nipple discharge, swelling, dimpling (retraction) of the nipple, or a lump that can be felt.

Early Diagnosis and Treatment Can Save Your Life

e

edema (e-de'-mah). Build-up of fluid in the tissues, resulting in swelling. Edema of the arm can occur after radical mastectomy, axillary dissection of lymph nodes, or radiation therapy, due to treatment or removal of the lymph channels. (Also see lymphedema.)

estrogen (es'-tre-jen). A female sex hormone produced primarily in the ovaries, possibly in the adrenal cortex, and produced in men in the testes (in much smaller amounts than in women). In women, levels of estrogen fluctuate on nature's carefully orchestrated schedule, regulating the development of secondary sex characteristics, including breasts; regulating the cycle of menstruation; and preparing the body for fertilization and reproduction. In breast cancer, estrogen may feed the growth of cancer cells.

estrogen receptor assay. A test to see if a breast tumor's cells are nourished by estrogen (estrogen-receptor positive) or not (estrogen-receptor negative). See also **progesterone receptor assay.**

estrogen replacement therapy. The use of estrogen (exogenous estrogen—i.e., estrogen not produced by the body; estrogen from other sources) to replace estrogen that the body would normally produce, but has ceased to produce because of natural or induced menopause. This type of hormone therapy is often prescribed to alleviate discomforts of menopause and has been shown to provide protective effects against heart disease and osteoporosis in post-menopausal women. Since estrogen nourishes some types of breast cancer, scientists are working on the question of whether estrogen replacement therapy increases breast cancer risk.

external radiation. Radiation therapy that uses a machine to aim high-energy rays at the cancer. Also called external beam radiation.

Early Diagnosis and Treatment Can Save Your Life

f

fibroadenoma. An adenoma in the breast composed of fibrous tissue. On clinical examination or breast self-examination, it feels like a firm lump. These usually occur in young women and are benign.

fibrocystic changes. A term that describes certain benign changes in the breast; also called fibrocystic disease or benign breast disease. Symptoms of this condition are breast swelling or pain. Signs that a physician can observe on clinical breast examination are the presence of nodularity (nodules), lumpiness, and sometimes, nipple discharge. Although these symptoms mimic breast cancer, microscopic examination of breast tissue shows that there is no cancer.

fine needle aspiration. See **needle aspiration.**

five-year survival. To survive cancer for five years after treatment of the disease. This is a "milestone" for most cancer patients, indicating that treatment was successful.

g

galactocele (gah-lak'to-sel). A clogged milk duct; a cyst filled with milk. It may occur in the breast during breastfeeding.

gene. A segment or unit of DNA that contains information on hereditary characteristics such as hair color, eye color, and height. Women who have the BRCA1 or BRCA2 gene have an inherited (genetic) tendency to develop breast cancer.

genetic. Related to the genes. See also **gene.**

generalized breast lumpiness. Breast irregularities and lumpiness, commonplace and non-cancerous. Sometimes called **fibrocystic disease** or **benign breast disease**.

Early Diagnosis and Treatment Can Save Your Life

grade. Cancer cells are graded by how much they look like normal cells. Grade 1 (also called well-differentiated) means the cancer cells look like the normal cells. Grade 3 (poorly differentiated) cancer cells do not look like normal cells at all. Grade 1 cancers aren't considered aggressive. In other words, they grow more slowly and metastasize slower. Grade 3 cancers are more likely to grow and metastasize faster. A cancer's grade along with its stage is used to determine treatment.

h

Halsted radical mastectomy. A type of surgery that removes the breast, skin, both pectoral muscles, and all axillary lymph nodes on the same site.

high risk. Having a higher risk of developing cancer, compared with the general population. Some of the factors that can place a person at high risk are heredity (a family history of breast cancer increases a risk of breast cancer), lifestyle changes (smoking increases risk of lung cancer), and the environment (exposure to sunlight increases risk of skin cancer). See also **risk factor**.

hormone. A chemical substance that is released into the body by the endocrine glands, such as the thyroid or ovaries. The substance travels through the bloodstream and sets in motion various body functions. For example, prolactin, which is produced in the pituitary gland, begins and sustains the production of milk in the breast after childbirth.

hormone receptor. A protein on the surface of a cell that binds to a specific hormone. The hormone cause many changes to take place in the cell.

hormone receptor assay. A test to see whether a breast tumor is likely to be affected by hormones or if it can be treated with hormones. (Also see **estrogen receptor assay, progesterone receptor assay.**)

Early Diagnosis and Treatment Can Save Your Life

hormone replacement therapy. Treatment that adds, locks, or removes hormones. For certain conditions (such as diabetes or menopause), hormones are given to adjust low hormone levels. To slow or stop the growth of certain cancers (such as prostate and breast cancer), synthetic hormones or other drugs may be given to block the body's natural hormones. Sometimes surgery is needed to remove the gland that makes a certain hormone. Also called hormonal therapy, hormone treatment, or endocrine therapy. (Also see **estrogen replacement therapy.**)

hyperplasia (hi''per-pla'ze-ah). An abnormal increase in the number of cells in a specific area, such as the lining of the breasts ducts. This overgrowth may be due to hormonal stimulation, injury, or continuous irritation. By itself, hyperplasia is not cancerous, but when the proliferating cells are atypical (unlike normal cells), the risk of cancer developing is greater.

i

immune system. The complex system by which the body resists invasion by a foreign substance such as bacterial infection or a transplanted organ. See **antibody, antigen.**

incisional biopsy. Surgical removal of a portion of an abnormal area or tissue or lump.

infiltrating ductal carcinoma. A cancer that starts in the milk passages (ducts) of the breast and then breaks through the duct wall, where it invades the fatty tissue of the breast. When it reaches this point, it has the potential to spread (metastasize) elsewhere in the breast, as well as to other parts of the body through the bloodstream and lymphatic system. Infiltrating ductal carcinoma is the most common type of breast cancer, accounting for about 80% of breast malignancies.

infraclavicular nodes. Lymph nodes located beneath the clavicle (collar bone); a part of the network of axillary lymph nodes.

Early Diagnosis and Treatment Can Save Your Life

in situ cancer. Very early or noninvasive growths that are confined to the ducts or lobules in the breast.

internal radiation. A procedure in which radioactive material sealed in needles, seeds, wires, or catheters is placed directly into or near a tumor. Also called brachytherapy, implant radiation, or interstitial radiation therapy.

interferon (in"ter-fer'on). A protein produced by cells, interferon helps regulate the body's immune system (immune response), boosting activity when a threat, such as a virus, is detected. Scientists have learned that interferon helps fight against cancer, so it is used with some chemotherapies and in bone marrow transplants. Interferon can be made artificially in large amounts.

internal mammary nodes. Lymph nodes located inside the chest next to the junction of the sternum (breastbone) and the ribs. The lymph glands of the breast drain into the internal mammary nodes.

intraductal papilloma (pap"i-lo'-mah). A small, finger-like, polyp-like benign tumor that starts in the ductal system of the breast. It can cause discharge from the nipple. Woman with papillomatosis (multiple intraductal papillomas) is at a slight increased risk of developing breast cancer.

invasive cancer. Cancer that has invaded surrounding tissue and spread to distant parts of the body.

invasive lobular (lob'u-lar) carcinoma. A cancer that arises in the milk-producing glands (lobules) of the breast and then breaks through the lobular walls. From this site, it may then spread elsewhere in the breast. About 15% of invasive breast cancers is invasive lobular carcinoma. It is often difficult to detect by physical examination or even by mammography. Up to 25% of women with this type of cancer will at some point develop an additional cancer in the opposite breast.

Early Diagnosis and Treatment Can Save Your Life

l

latissmus dorsi flap procedure. A method of breast reconstruction that uses the long flat muscle of the back, by rotating it to the chest area.

lobular carcinoma *in situ*. A very early type of breast cancer that develops within the milk-producing glands (lobules) of the breast and does not penetrate through the walls of the lobules. Researchers think that lobular carcinoma *in situ* does not eventually become an invasive lobular cancer; however, having this type of cancer places a woman at increased risk of developing an invasive breast cancer later in life. For this reason, it's important for women with lobular carcinoma *in situ* to have a physical examination three or four times a year and an annual mammogram.

lobular carcinoma (infiltrating or invasive). A type of breast cancer that starts within the lobules. It may be multicentric (occurring in multiple lobules). Compared with other types of breast cancer, this type has a higher chance of occurring in the opposite breast, as well. It can often be difficult to diagnose, even with careful physical examination or mammography.

lobules. The milk-producing parts of the breast located at one end of the ducts. The nipple is located at the opposite end of the ducts.

localization biopsy. (Also known as needle localization.) Using mammography or ultrasound to locate an area of concern that cannot be felt by hand.

localized breast cancer. A cancer that arose in the breast and is confined to the breast.

lump. Any kind of mass that can be felt in the breast or elsewhere in the body.

Early Diagnosis and Treatment Can Save Your Life

lumpectomy (lum-pek'to-me). Surgery to remove the tumor and a small amount of surrounding normal tissue. See also **mastectomy, two-step procedure.**

lymph nodes. Small masses of bean-shaped tissue, located along the lymphatic vessels, that remove waste and fluids from lymph and act as filters of impurities in the body.

lymphatic system. The tissues and organs (including bone marrow, spleen, thymus, and lymph nodes) that produce and store lymphocytes (cells that fight infection) and the channels that carry the lymph fluid. The entire lymphatic system is an important part of the body's immune system.

lymphedema (lim"fe-de'mah). Swelling in the arm caused by excess fluid that collects in the lymph nodes and vessels are removed by surgery or treated by radiation. This condition is usually painful and can be persistent.

lymphoma. Tumor made up of lymph node tissue, from an abnormal production of immature lymphocytes (a form of white blood cells). About 5% of all cancers are lymphomas. One form is Hodgkin's disease. Lymphoma can occur as a result of some types of cancer therapies.

m

malignant tumor. A mass of cancer cells that may invade surrounding tissues or spread (metastasize) to distant areas of the body. See **cancer.**

mammogram, mammography. An x-ray of the breast; the principal method of detecting breast cancer in women over 40. Mammography is performed on a special type of x-ray machine that is used only for this purpose. It has two plates. The lower plate is metal and has a drawer for the film cassette. The bare breast is placed on this plate. The upper plate, which is clear plastic, is lowered onto the breast. Thus compressed, it is possible to obtain a clear image of the interior structures of the breast (mammogram). The compression is maintained for only a few seconds, long enough for the tech-

Early Diagnosis and Treatment Can Save Your Life

nician to go to the control panel and snap the image. The procedure is then repeated with the other breast. A mammogram can show a developing breast tumor before it is large enough to be felt by a woman or even by a highly skilled health professional.

mammaplasty. Plastic surgery to reconstruct the breast or to change the shape, size, or position of the breast. Reduction mammaplasty reduces the size of the breast. Augmentation mammaplasty enlarges a woman's breast, usually with implants.

margin. The normal tissue around a tumor. Positive means there is cancer at the margin or the margin is less than 1mm. More than 1mm is negative margin. If the margin is positive, more surgery may be done to make it negative.

mastectomy (mas-tek'to-me). Surgery to remove all or part of the breast. *Extended radical mastectomy* removes the breast, skin, pectoral muscles (both major and minor), and all axillary and internal mammary lymph nodes on the same side. *Modified radical mastectomy* removes the breast, skin, both pectoral muscles, and all axillary lymph nodes on the same side, leaving the chest muscles intact. *Partial mastectomy* removes less than the whole breast, taking only part of the breast in which the cancer occurs and a margin of health breast tissue surrounding the tumor. See also **lumpectomy**. *Prophylactic mastectomy* is removal of the interior of one or both breasts, before any evidence of cancer can be found, for the purpose of preventing cancer. This procedure is sometimes recommended for women at very high risk of breast cancer, but its efficacy is not proven. *Quadrantectomy* is a partial mastectomy in which the quarter of the breast that contains a tumor is removed. *Segmented mastectomy* is a partial mastectomy. *Simple mastectomy* is a term once used to describe what is now called total mastectomy. *Total mastectomy* removes only the breast.

mastitis. Inflammation or infection of the breast.

Early Diagnosis and Treatment Can Save Your Life

medullary carcinoma. A special type of infiltrating breast cancer in which the tumor appears well-defined, with obvious boundaries between tumor tissue and normal tissue. About 5% of breast cancers are medullary carcinomas. The outlook (prognosis) for this kind of cancer is considered to be better than average.

menopause. The time in a woman's life when monthly cycles of menstruation stop forever and the level of hormones produced by the ovaries decreases. Menopause usually naturally occurs in a woman's late 40's or early 50's, but it can also be caused by surgical removal of both ovaries, or by chemotherapy, which often destroys ovarian function.

metastasis. The spread of cancer cells to distant areas of the body by way of the lymph system or bloodstream.

modified radical mastectomy. A type of breast cancer surgery that removes the breast, skin, nipple, areola, and most of the axillary lymph nodes on the same side, leaving the chest muscles intact.

n

needle aspiration. Removal of fluid from a cyst, or cells from a tumor. In this procedure, a needle and syringe (like those used to give injections) is used to pierce the skin, reach the cyst or tumor, and with suction, draw up (aspirate) specimens for biopsy analysis. If the needle is thin, the procedure is called fine needle aspiration or "FNA." If a needle with a large bore (or core) is used, the procedure is called a **core biopsy.**

needle biopsy. See **needle aspiration.**

needle localization biopsy. A procedure used to do a breast needle biopsy when the lump is difficult to locate or in areas that look suspicious on the x-ray but do not have a distinct lump. After an injection of local anethesia to numb the area, a thin needle is inserted in the breast.

Early Diagnosis and Treatment Can Save Your Life

X-rays are taken and used to guide the wire to the area to be biopsied. A tiny hook on the end of the wire holds it in place. Then a hypodermic needle (like the type used to give injections) is injected, using the path of the wire as a guide, and the biopsy is completed. See also **needle aspiration**.

nipple. The tip of the breast; the pigmented projection in the middle of the areola. The nipple contains the opening of milk ducts from the breast.

nipple discharge. Any fluid coming from the nipple. It may be clear, milky, bloody, tan, gray or green.

nodal status. A count of the number of lymph nodes in the armpit (axillary nodes) to which cancer has spread (node positive) or has not spread (node-negative). The number and site of positive axillary nodes help forecast the risk of cancer recurrence.

node. Lymph glands.
nodule. A small, solid lump that can be located by touch.

noncancerous. Benign; not malignant; no cancer is present.

normal hormonal changes. Changes in breast and other tissues that are caused by fluctuation in levels of female hormones during the menstrual cycle.

nurse practitioner. A nurse who has completed the RN (registered nurse) degree and then takes highly specialized training. Nurse practitioners can work with or without the supervision of a physician. They take on additional duties in diagnosis and treatment of patients and in many states they may write prescriptions.

Early Diagnosis and Treatment Can Save Your Life

o

oncologist (on-col'o-gist). A doctor who is specially trained in the diagnosis and treatment of cancer. *Medical Oncologists* specialize in the use of drugs and/or chemotherapy to treat cancer. *Radiation Oncologists* specialize in the use of x-rays (radiation) to kill tumors. Medical and radiation oncologists often cooperate in giving complicated treatments.

one-step procedure. Surgery in which a breast treatment (such as a mastectomy, if the diagnosis is indeed breast cancer) is performed in a single operation. The patient is given general anesthesia and does not know until awakened if the diagnosis was cancer or surgery was performed. Once the only option in breast cancer, the one-step procedure is now rarely used.

p

Paget's disease of the nipple. A form of breast cancer that begins in the milk passages (ducts) and involves the skin of the nipple and areola. A sign of Paget's disease is a crusting, scaly, red, inflamed tissue (dermatitis) lesion of the nipple. With true Paget's disease, cancer is usually also present within the breast. This is a rare type of cancer that occurs in 1% of cases. If no lump can be felt, it generally has a good outcome (prognosis).

palliative (pal'e-a"-tiv) treatment. Therapy that relieves symptoms, such as pain, but does not cure the disease. Its main purpose is to improve the quality of live. The use of chemotherapy to shrink more advanced cancer tumors when curing the cancer is not possible.

palpation. A simple technique using the hands to examine the surface of the body to feel the organs and tissue underneath. A palpable mass in the breast is one that can be felt.

Early Diagnosis and Treatment Can Save Your Life

partial mastectomy. A form of breast cancer surgery that removes less than the whole breast, taking only part of the breast in which the cancer occurs and a margin of healthy breast tissue surrounding the tumor (Also see **lumpectomy**.)

pathologist (pa-thol'o-gist). A physician who specializes in the identification of abnormalities and disease by examining body tissue under a microscope and organs. The pathologist determines whether a lump is benign or cancerous.

pathology (pa-thol'o-ji). The study of disease. Examination of body tissues and organs under a microscope for evidence of disease. Any tumor thought to be cancer must be diagnosed by examination under a microscope.

pectoral (pek'-tor-al) muscles. Muscles attached to the front of the chest wall and upper arms. The larger group is called *pectoralis major* and a smaller group is called *pectoralis minor*. Because these muscles are in close proximity to the breast, they may become involved in breast cancer or surgery to treat it.

pigment. A class of substances that provide color, including in the human body. The areola and nipple of the breast are pigmented with melanin. Normally a brownish tint, melanin in these areas of the breast can range from pale pink to deep brown.

placebo (plah-se'bo). An inert, inactive substance, sometimes called a "sugar pill." A placebo may be used in clinical trials to compare the effects of a given treatment against no treatment.

precancerous. See **malignant**.

predisposition. Susceptibility to a disease that can be triggered under certain conditions. For example, some women have a family history of breast cancer and are therefore predisposed (but not necessarily destined) to develop breast cancer.

Early Diagnosis and Treatment Can Save Your Life

premalignant. Abnormal changes in cells that may, but not always, become cancer. Most of these early lesions respond well to treatment and result in cure. Also called **precancerous.**

prevention. Avoiding the occurrence of an event, such as development of cancer, by avoiding things known to cause cancer and participating in activities that can or might prevent cancer. For example, avoiding smoking can prevent lung cancer, and taking Tamoxifen may prevent breast cancer in women who are at high risk for the disease.

primary cancer. The site where cancer begins. Primary cancer is usually named after the organ in which it starts (for example, breast cancer).

progesterone (pro-jes'-te-ron). A female sex hormone released by the ovaries during menstrual cycle to prepare the uterus for pregnancy and the breasts for milk production (lactation).

progesterone receptor assay. A test that shows whether a breast cancer depends on progesterone for growth. Progesterone receptors are tested along with estrogen receptors for more complete information on the hormone sensitivity of a cancer, and how best to treat it. See also **estrogen receptor.**

prognosis. A prediction of the course of disease or the outlook for the cure of the patient. For example, women with breast cancer that was detected early and received prompt treatment have a good prognosis.

proliferating. Multiplying or increasing in number. In biology, cell proliferation occurs by a process known as cell division.

prophylactic mastectomy. Women at very high risk of breast cancer may elect prophylactic (preventive) mastectomy. This is an operation in which one or both breasts are removed before there is a known breast cancer.

prosthesis. An artificial form, such as a breast prosthesis, that can be worn under the clothing after a mastectomy. (Plural: **prostheses**).

Early Diagnosis and Treatment Can Save Your Life

r

radiation oncologist. See **Oncologist.**

radical (Halsted or standard) mastectomy. See **mastectomy.**

radiologist (ra'di-ol'o-gist). A physician who has taken additional years of training to produce and read x-rays and other types of images (for example, ultrasound or magnetic resonance imaging [MRI]) for the purpose of diagnosing abnormalities.

Reach to Recovery. A visitation program of the American Cancer Society for women who have a personal concern about breast cancer. Carefully selected and trained volunteers who have successfully adjusted to breast cancer and its treatment provide information and support to women newly diagnosed with the disease.

rectus abdominus flap procedure. A method of breast reconstruction in which tissue from the lower abdominal wall which receives its blood supply from the rectus abdominus muscle, is used. The tissue from this area is moved up to the chest to create a breast mound and usually does not require an implant. Moving muscle and tissue from the lower abdomen to the chest results in flattening of the lower abdomen. Also called a TRAM flap.

recurrence. Cancer that has re-occurred, or reappeared after treatment. *Local recurrence* is at the same site as the original cancer. *Metastasis* means that the cancer has recurred at a distant site. *Regional recurrence* is in the lymph nodes near the site.

red blood cells. Red blood cells (also called erythrocytes) serve two important functions. With the help of an iron-containing protein called *hemoglobin*, they carry oxygen from the lungs to cells in all parts of the body. Oxygen helps cells obtain energy from the nutrients we eat. RBCs also take carbon dioxide back to the lungs from the cells; carbon dioxide is released as a waste product of cell processes. Too few blood cells

Early Diagnosis and Treatment Can Save Your Life

or too little hemoglobin is a condition known as *anemia*. It can cause weakness, lack of energy, dizziness, shortness of breath, headache, and irritability.

remission. Complete or partial disappearance of the signs and symptoms of cancer in response to treatment; the period in which a disease is under control. A remission may not be a cure.

replacement hormone therapy. See **estrogen replacement therapy.**

risk factor. Anything that increases a person's chance of getting a disease, such as cancer. The known risk factors for breast cancer are: family history of the disease, especially in one's mother or sister; beginning menstrual periods at an early age (before age 12); obesity; never having completed a pregnancy; first pregnancy after age 30.

S

saline breast implant. A breast implant that is filled with saline solution.

saline solution. Saltwater solution.

screening. The search for disease, such as cancer, in people without symptoms. Screening may refer to coordinated programs in large populations. The principal screening measure for breast cancer is mammography.

side effects. After-effects or secondary effects of treatment, such as hair loss caused by chemotherapy and fatigue caused by radiation therapy.

silicone gel. Synthetic gel compound used in breast implants because of its flexibility, strength, and texture, which is similar to the texture of the natural breast. Silicone gel implants are available for women who have had breast cancer surgery, but only under the auspices of a clinical trial. See also **breast implant.**

Early Diagnosis and Treatment Can Save Your Life

simple mastectomy. A form of breast cancer surgery used to describe what is now called total mastectomy.

staging. A method of determining and describing the extent of cancer, based on the size of the tumor, whether regional axillary lymph nodes are involved, and whether distant spread (metastasis) has occurred. Knowing the stage at diagnosis helps decide the best treatment and the prognosis:

Stage 0	The earliest type of breast cancer; the disease is *in situ* and has not spread within or beyond the breast.
Stage 1	The tumor is less than one inch in diameter and has not spread beyond the breast.
Stage 2	The tumor is about one to two inches in diameter, and may or may not have spread to the lymph nodes under the arm (axillary lymph nodes).
Stage 3	The tumor is about two inches or larger in diameter, and has spread to the axillary lymph nodes, and/or to other lymph nodes, or to other tissues near the breast.
Stage 4	The cancer has spread (metastasized) to other organs of the body.

stem cells. The cells from which all blood cells develop.

stereotactic (ste"-re-o-tak'tik) core needle biopsy. A method of needle biopsy that is useful in some cases in which a mass can be seen on a mammogram but cannot be located by touch. Computerized equipment maps the location of the mass and this is used as a guide for the placement of the needle. See also **needle aspiration**.

systemic chemotherapy. Treatment with anti-cancer drugs that travel through the blood to cells all over the body.

Early Diagnosis and Treatment Can Save Your Life

t

Tamoxifen (tah-moks'i-fen) - brand name: Nolvadex. A drug that blocks estrogen; an antiestrogen drug. Blocking estrogen is desirable in some cases of breast cancer because estrogen feeds the growth of certain types of tumors. This drug is being tested in a large clinical trial to see if it will help prevent the recurrence of cancer.

TRAM flap. Uses tissue taken from the woman's abdomen. The surgery is complicated and time-consuming, adding many hours to a mastectomy operation when the reconstruction is immediate. A section of skin, underlying fat, and a portion of abdominal muscle is excised, leaving one or two pedicles of tissue with the natural blood supply. The flap is tunneled under the abdominal wall to the chest and rotated to fit the mastectomy wound.

tumor. Tissue growth in which the cells multiply uncontrollably; also called **neoplasm**. Can be either benign or malignant.

two-step procedure. A method in which breast biopsy for diagnosis and breast surgery for treatment (i.e., lumpectomy or mastectomy, if the diagnosis is indeed breast cancer) are performed as two separate procedures, after an interval of days or weeks. This method is strongly preferred by women and their health care team because it allows time to consider all options.

u

ultrasonography. An imaging method in which high-frequency sound waves are used to outline a part of the body. High-frequency sound waves are transmitted through the area of the body being studied. The sound wave echoes are picked up and displayed on a television screen. This painless method is used mainly to find out if a structure is solid or liquid. It is useful in detecting breast cysts in young women with firm, fibrous breasts. No radiation exposure occurs. Also called **ultrasound.**

Early Diagnosis and Treatment Can Save Your Life

unilateral. Affecting one side of the body. For example, unilateral breast cancer occurs in one breast only.

W

white blood cells. A name for several types of cells in blood that remain after red cells have been removed. Their purpose is to help defend against infection. T-cell lymphocytes and B-cell lymphocytes are two types of white blood cells that play a role in the immune system against cancer. They function by destroying "foreign" substances such as bacteria and viruses. When an infection is present, their production increases. If the number of leukocytes (white blood cells) is abnormally low (a condition known as *leukopenia*), infection is more likely to occur, and it is more difficult for the body to rid itself of the infection.

X

x-rays. One form of radiation that can, at low levels, produce an image of cancer on film, and at high levels, can destroy cancer cells.

Early Diagnosis and Treatment Can Save Your Life

*If God brings you to it,
He'll bring you through it.
In happy moments, praise God.
In difficult moments, seek God.
In quiet moments, worship God.
In painful moments, trust God.
Every moment, thank God.*

Author Unknown

In memory of the women and men who have lost their lives to this disease.

RESOURCES & REFERENCES

<u>AMERICAN CANCER SOCIETY (ACS) PUBLICATIONS</u>
Breast Cancer Facts and Figures 2003-2004, No. 8610.03
Facts On Breast Cancer, No. 2003-LE
Cancer Facts & Figures for African Americans 2003-2004, No. 8614.03
Breast Cancer – No. 9405-06
Breast Self-Examination – A New Approach, No. 6438.39
Mastectomy: A Patient Guide, No. 4600
Common Breasts Conditions, No. 9710
Talking To Your Doctor, No. 4638-PS
Breast Reconstruction After Mastectomy, No. 4650
American With Disabilities Act, No. 4571
Chemotherapy What It Is, How It Helps, No. 4512
Breast Cancer Dictionary, No. 4675
For Women Facing Breast Cancer, No. 4652
If You've Thought About Breast Cancer, No. 4627
Breast Cancer (Treatment Guidelines for Patients), No. 9405.06
Women's Health & Cancer Rights Acts

<u>NATIONAL CANCER INSTITUTE</u> (National Institute of Health)
What You Need to Know About Breast Cancer, No. 95-1556
Understanding Breast Changes (A Guide For All Women), No.96-3536
Questions and Answers About Breast Lumps, No. 93-2401
Get The Facts – What Is Complementary and Alternative Medicine (CAM)
General Information About Male Breast Cancer
Male Breast Cancer – Treatment Option Overview

<u>POSITIVE PROMOTIONS</u>
Women & Breast Health (Item No.KLT-4)
  • Breast Changes That Need Attention

<u>KRAMES-STAYWELL</u>
Breast Health, Item No. 1349
   • Looking in From The Outside
   • What You Feel
Breast Lumps, Item No. 1019
   • The Simple 1-2-3 of Breast Self-Examination (text only)
Breast Surgery, Item No. 1291
   • A Mammogram

WEBSITES WORTH VISITING
www.acs.org
www.aabcainc@yahoo.com
www.alternative-cancer-treatments.com
www.annieappleseedproject.org
www.avoncompany.com
www.bwwla.com
www.breastcancerfund.org
www.bcresource.org
www.cancer.org
www.canceradvocacy.org
www.cancercare.org
www.cancer.gov
www.cdc.gov
www.celebratinglife.org
www.gildasclub.org
www.johnwnickfoundation.org
www.komen.org
www.natlbcc.org
www.nccam.nih.gov
www.ods.odod.nih.gov
www.plasticsurgery.org
www.prevention.com
www.sharecancersupport.org
www.sisternetworkinc.org
www.thebreastsite.com
www.winabc.org
www.youngsurvival.org
www.y-me.org
www.4women.gov

SCRIPTURES TAKEN FROM THE HOLY BIBLE, KING JAMES VERSION
Psalm 139:14
Psalm 57:1
Jeremiah 30:17
Deuteronomy 31:6
James 1:3
2 Corinthians 12:9
Isaiah 40:31

INDEX

A

ACS (American Cancer Society), 150, 231, 239
    clinical trials matching service, 182, 210
    recommendations for examinations, 154
acupuncture, 178
ADA (Americans With Disabilities Act), 222
adjuvant therapy, 168-169, 172-174
    side effects of, 173-174
aerola, reconstruction of, 192
age and breast cancer, 124, 125, 136, 154, 196
alcohol, 195
alternative medicine. see specific terms, 176-181
American Board of Medical Specialists, 161
American Society of Clinical Oncology, 161
American Society of Plastic Surgeons, 162
anatomy, of breasts, 131-132, 133
changes in, 135-136
in males, 213
anti-estrogen (Tamoxifen), 174-175
aromatherapy, 178
artificial breast, 185-186,
Ask-A-Nurse, 161
aspiration, 163, 165
    fine needle, 164
autologous breast reconstruction
    benefits, 189
    complications, 191
    types, 190-191

axillary lymph node dissection, 171
Ayurveda, 178

B

biopsy
    core needle, 164
    questions about, 202-203
    types of, 163-165
blood tests, 151
bone scan, 151
bra, wearing, 127
    and prosthesis, 186
BRCA1 and BRCA2 genes, 151-152, 171, 182-183
breast
    changes in, 156
    size, 128, 195
    specialist, 161-162
breast-feeding, 129
BSE (breast self-examination), 142-146, *143, 144, 145, 146, 198*
    performing, 198

C

CAD (computer-aided diagnosis), 152
calcifications, 138-139
CAM (complementary and alternative medicine), 176-181
cancer, breast
    carcinoma, types, 158
    causation, 182-183
    defined, 157
    general questions, 203-204
    inflammatory breast, 158, 160

issues after diagnosis, 203-204
Tamoxifen and risk, 175
recurrence of, 161
risk factors for, 194-196, 214
stages of, 159-161
types of, 157-158, 214
carcinoma, types. see also cancer, 158
causation, 129, 182-183, 196
chemotherapy, 172-174, 206-207
for men, 215-216
high-dose, 174
myths about, 129
questions to ask, 206-207
side effects, 173-174
chest x-ray, 151
Chinese medicine, traditional, 181
chiropractic, 179
clinical trials, 181-182, 216
questions about, 210
complementary medicine. see specific terms, 176-181
complications
in reconstruction, 191
computer tomography, 151
conditions, breast, 136-140
costochronditis, 139-140
CT scan, 151
cysts, 137
aspirating, 163

D

deodorant use, 127
detection. *see also* mammogram, 151-154
dietary supplements, 179
drug
Tamoxifen, 174-175
trials, 181-182

E

electric blankets, 129

EMF (electromagnetic fields), 179
exam, breast
and woman's age, 154
clinical, 153-154
self-, 142-146
excisional biopsy, 163-164
exercise, 185, 195
external beam radiation, 172

F

facts, general, 123, 194-196
Family and Medical Leave Act, 223-224
fat necrosis, 138
fat, in foods, 127, 185
Federal Rehabilitation Act, 223
fibroadenoma, 137-138
fibrocystic breast changes, 137
finances, 226
government help for, 226
insurance, 197, 225
fine needle aspiration, 164
free flap, 191
complications of, 191

G

genetic factors, 124, 151-152, 181-182
genetic testing, 181-182
glossary, 241-268

H

Halsted Radical, 170
HER-2-neu, 153
high-dose chemotherapy, 174
hormone receptor testing, 152
hormone therapy
for men, 216
questions to ask about, 210
hormones
as risk factor, 195, 197

I

in situ cancers, 157
incisional biopsy, 164
infection, of breast, 139
inflammatory breast cancer, 158, 160
insurance, 197, 225
    finding mammogram without, 150
    NCCS pamphlet, 225
    post-treatment, 227-229
    Women's Health Act, 220-221
integrative medicine, 177
intraductal papillomas, 138
invasive cancers, 157-158

L

legislation
    ADA (Americans With Disabilities Act), 222
    Family and Medical Leave Act, 223-224
    Federal Rehabilitation Act, 223
    Patients' Bill of Rights and Responsibilities, 218-219
    state, 223
    WHCRA (Women's Health and Cancer Rights Act), 220-221
localization biopsy, 165
lump, 156
    actions after discovery of, 162-166, 201
    benign, 136-137
    illustrated, 142
    lumpectomy, 170
        pain and, 197
        questions to ask about, 201
        steps to take after finding, 162-166
lumpectomy, 169
lymph node
    surgery for, 171
lymphedema, 183

M

males, breast cancer in, 126, 213-216
    and Tamoxifen, 175
    survival, 216
    treatment options, 215-216
mammary duct ectasia, 139
mammograms, 149
    age and, 148, 196
    digital, 152
    emotions surrounding, 199-200
    low-cost, 150
    myths about, 127-128, 128
    questions about, 199-200, 200
massage, 179
mastectomy
    Halsted Radical, 170
    modified radical, 170
    partial, 170
    prophylactic, 170-171
    radical, 170
    side effects after, 183
    simple, 170
medical team, 168
medical oncologist, 161
medicine
    alternative, 176-181
    Chinese, 181
    menopause, 136
menstrual cycle, 135
MRI (magnetic resonance imaging), 152
myths, 124-129
    about mammograms, 128
    causation, 129

N

National Cancer Institute, 150, 161, 216
naturopathic, 179-180
NCCAM (National Center for Complementary and Alternative Medicine)
    classifications, 177-178
needle biopsy, 164
needle localization, 165
nipple

changes in, 156
discharge, 139, 156
nipple/areola reconstruction, 192
Nolvadex, 174-175
nutrition, 185, 195
    dietary supplements, 179
    fat in foods, xxx

O

oncologist, 168
oral contraceptives, 195, 197
orange-peel skin, 156, 158
organizations. *See also under* specific names, 231-238
osteopathic, 180

P

Patients Bill of Rights and Repsonsibilities, 218-219
PET (positron emission tomography), 152
pregnancy, 135-136
PRO (peer review organizations), 227-229
prognosis, for men, 216
prostheses, 185-186
puberty, 135

Q

qi-gong, 180

R

race. and cancer, 126
radiation therapy, 169, 171-172, 205-206
    for men, 216
    questions to ask, 205-206
reconstruction, breast
    autologous, 189-190
    complications to, 191
    free flap, 191
    general questions, 208-209

    nipple/areola, 192
    questions to ask, 207-108, 207-109
    TRAM flap, 190
recurrence, 161
    treatment for, 184-192
reiki, 180
resources, 271-272
risk factors, 124
    in males, 214
    reducing, 196

S

safety, of mammograms, 128
scan
    bone, 151
    CT, 151
sclerosing adenosis, 138
side effects
    of chemotherapy, 173-174
smoking, 195
sonogram, 153
sores, breast, 156
specialists, medical, 168
stages, of breast cancer, 159-161
stereotactic localization biopsy, 165
support
    from family, 211-212
    groups, 231-238
surgery, breast
    autologous reconstruction, 189-191
    for men, 215
    free flap, 191
    general questions, 209
    implants, 187-189
    questions to ask, 209
    reconstruction, 189-192
    TRAM flap, 190

T

Tamoxifen, 174-175
    side effects of, 175
TCM (traditional Chinese medicine), 181
testing, genetic, 181-182
tests, blood, 151
therapeutic touch, 180
therapy
    adjuvant, 172-174
    alternative, 176-180
    alternative medical systems, 177
    bioelectromagnetic-based, 178
    biofield, 178
    biologically based, 177
    chemo-, 172-174, 206-207
    clinical trials for new, 181-182
    energy, 178
    hormonal, 174-175, 210
    lymphedema as side effect to, 183
    manipulative, 177-178
    mind-body intervention, 177
    radiation, 171-172, 205-206
    transplantation
    bone marrow, 176
    stem cell, 175-176
TRAM (transverse rectus abdominous muscle) flap, 190
transplantation
    bone marrow, 176
    stem cell, 175-176
treatment
    biopsy, 163-165
    follow-up to, 184-192
    lumpectomy, 169
    mastectomy, 170
    primary alternatives, 169-171
    radiation therapy, 171-172
    specialists for, 167-169
trials, clinical, 181-182

U

ultrasound, 153

W

warning signs, 156
weight fluctuation, 136
WHCRA (Women's Health and Cancer Rights Act), 220-221
workplace issues, 223-224
    ADA, 222
    government regulations and, 223

Y

YWCA Encore Plus Program, 150, 238

About the Author

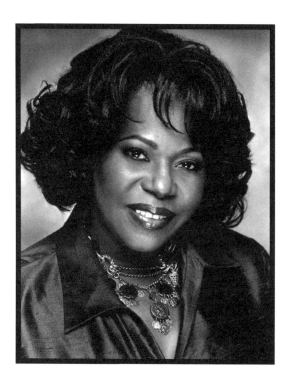

M. Nicole Bryant was born in St. Louis, Missouri and raised in East Carondelet, Illinois where she currently resides. She attended Southern Illinois University in Edwardsville before moving to Oakland, California. Her diagnosis propelled her into a life of breast cancer advocacy and awareness. Her passion in life is to educate and inform women, particularly women of color, of the importance of taking a proactive role in their health care. Her mission is to help women (and men) cope with the challenges that such a diagnosis brings and help them understand that early detection and treatment is one of the keys to survival. She has taken her message of hope, faith, and empowerment everywhere from prisons to churches. Her accomplishments include:

- Member, Chairmaine Chapman Society of the United Way, (2003 - Current)
- Honoree, National Council of Negro Women, Inc., Ethele Scott Section, East St. Louis, IL, February 2006

- Honorary Chairperson, American Cancer Society's 2005 Relay For Life, East St. Louis Chapter, July 2005
- Honoree, Top Ladies of Distinction (East St. Louis Chapter) "Women of Courage" Who Through It All... Keep The Faith, April 2005
- Reach To Recover Volunteer, American Cancer Society (ACS)
- Certified "Special Touch" Best Health Facilitator, American Cancer Society
- Volunteer, Women's Cancer Research Center, Berkeley, California
- Guest speaker, facilitator, and assisted in the coordination of numerous breast cancer workshops, conferences, and tasks force. These include:
    - Kaiser Hospital, Oakland, CA
    - Alameda County's Early Detection Program - Speaker's Bureau
    - Peralta Community College District Series, Oakland, CA
    - West Oakland Health Center, Oakland, CA
    - Sisters For Positive Change (Mills College), Oakland, CA
    - A Turning Point, San Rafael, California
    - Alta Bates Hospital Comprehensive Breast Cancer Center
    - Department of Energy's Federally Employed Women, Oakland, CA
    - Contra Costa County Division of Corrections, Richmond, CA
    - Guest speaker at numerous churches and community organizations throughout Oakland, CA
- Author - "Breast Reconstruction and Body Image"
- Performed in "Art Rages Us", San Francisco, CA - Breast Cancer From 8 to 80, 1998
- Featured in ABC TV News Segment, (Channel 7, San Francisco/Oakland, CA), October 1997 - "Breast Cancer: Beating The Odds", 1997

**Ms. Bryant is available for speaking engagements.
You may contact her at nbryant@htc.net or 618-286-3648**

How To Order

Copies may be purchased through
Precisely Write Publishing
P. O. Box 411
East Carondelet, IL 62240
Telephone: 618-286-3648
Fax: 618-286-4026

Quantity discounts are also available.

Visit our website at: www.breastlessness.com